Quandaries:

Understanding Mental Illnesses in Persons with Developmental Disabilities

Sue Gabriel

Quandaries: Understanding Mental Illnesses in Persons with Developmental Disabilities

Sue Gabriel

Copyright © 2004 NADD Press

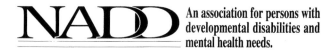

An association for persons with developmental disabilities and mental health needs.

132 Fair Street
Kingston, New York 12401

LCCN: 2004110133
ISBN: 1-57256-041-X

1st Printing 2004

Printed in the United States of America

Contents

Dedication

Mom? MOM!? <u>M M O O M M</u>!!

To my family, for all the times I was
buried in thought at the computer. Thanks for your
support, understanding, and most of all love.

Disclaimer Statement

In the writing and updating of this text, the author has made every
attempt to provide current relevant data. As new information is always
coming out, however, this book is to be used as a guide/primer, not a
substitute for appropriate diagnosis and treatment from trained professionals. This book provides general guides, but each person must be
assessed as the unique individual that they are.

Chapter 1

In the Beginning

Job 38:2b
"...words without knowledge."

My first paid job in the field of disabilities . . . assuming one calls a $1.85 an hour "paid" . . . was at an adult foster care home in northern Michigan. I was eighteen years old. My orientation consisted of, "Here's the stove, refrigerator, 20 people, and we pass these pills out at lunch time." Living in this home were two elderly brothers Henry and Tom. Besides being brothers, they looked a lot alike for other reasons. They both had large, protruding, low set ears. They both had thin, elongated faces. While it was my first lesson in genetics, I certainly didn't understand its importance at the time. As a typical High School graduate, I was sure I already knew all of life's secrets. On this routine summer day at the group home, however, I would learn many things when Tom wouldn't come down for lunch.

Ever have one of those days when everything goes wrong? The first lesson of the day involved making soup. A typical lunch in this group home consisted of sandwiches and soup. The soup was made from canned vegetable soup or cream of mushroom soup and I was to throw in whatever leftovers were left over from the refrigerator. (Needless to say, this was before the days of pre-written, nutritionist approved menus.) I learned that one should *never, ever* add canned beets to cream of anything soup, or you get putrid pink soup as a result. I also learned that one shouldn't yell at one's boss when some members of the household won't come down for lunch.

In between these lessons, I learned that one should never place their shins within kicking range when Tom is wearing nothing (and I mean nothing) but steel-toed work boots. It would be many years before I would realize that Tom and Henry provided me with some of my first lessons in not only genetics, but also the often-complicated world of dual diagnosis.

Tom and Henry had been diagnosed with severe mental retardation early in life. In 1926 at the ages of five and six respectively, they were placed in an institution because their "out of control" behaviors made it impossible for the family to care for them alone. Their retardation allowed the schools to refuse them services. Suspecting something familial (genetics being almost unknown), their sister opted to never marry, nor to have children. Although she remained faithful as their guardian and loved them until the very end of their lives, she had concerns. In addition to her brothers, two out of three uncles, and several male cousins all had similar facial features and levels of disabilities. She herself had gone on to college and was a university professor until retirement, but several of her female cousins were similarly affected as the males but to a lesser extent.

What she suspected as something familial, but was not understood even in the late 1970's when I worked in this home, was the nature of Fragile X. Fragile X is considered to be the number one inherited disorder causing mental retardation particularly in males. It is associated with autism spectrum disorders, hand flapping, avoidant eye gaze, elongated faces, and bodies, and abnormally large testicles (in males). As her brothers aged, Henry became more placid and easygoing and indeed was the perfect couch potato. As Tommy aged, however, his tolerance for change, tolerance for others, indeed his tolerance for much of anything decreased dramatically.

On this warm summer day in a home built long before the wonders of air conditioning, it must have been too warm for clothes — at least for Tom. Why he kept on steel-toed work boots, I do not know. What my pre-1980's high school biology text never informed me (enlarged external genitalia), I was about to learn. I could not determine which was worse — the cream of beet soup, or my reaction as I recognized Tom had no clothes on.

While everyone else was politely eating the putrid pink soup (Rex who was blind and liked beets, thought it tasted good!), Tom was upstairs screaming. I went upstairs to convince him that: a.) Clothes are necessary in the presence of everyone else. b.) the putrid pink soup wasn't that bad and, c.) please stop screaming, my head hurt. Tom wasn't willing to buy even one out of the three of these.

Tom aimed those size 12 steel-toed boots at my shins with remarkable accuracy. I beat (no pun intended) a hasty retreat. When I got back downstairs, I discovered everyone but Rex (who was still asking for seconds) trying to feed his or her soup to the dog. My boss asked why Tom wasn't eating. In rather impolite language, I let it be known that I didn't know and furthermore didn't care. I almost quit that day. In spite of all my goof-ups and likely because even then it was hard to find reasonable help for $1.85 an hour, my boss calmed me down and I stayed. Tom's difficulties however continued.

At this point in the late 1970's, even behaviorism hadn't quite made its way to the northern wilds of Michigan. Unfortunately the usage of Vitamin M (Mellaril) and Vitamin H (Haldol) had. Their use, or misuse, to tranquilize out just about any unwanted behavior was used with alarming frequency. Understanding of syndromes, and most certainly of psychiatric disorders in persons with developmental disabilities was nonexistent. It would take me many more years to think of the questions (trust me, I was GLAD to give Tom his Vitamin M since I thought it would calm him down), much less come to an understanding of dual diagnosis. On the other hand, the lesson of the steel-toed boots and the putrid pink soup would live on forever.

In my many years of working with people who have a developmental disability and co-morbid psychiatric impairments, I have been often criticized or acclaimed for commenting on the labels that one must use. Older labels of disabilities included such terms as imbecile, high or low-grade moron, and mentally defective. The more current labels of mild, moderate, severe and profound mental retardation are often not any better. In psychiatry, labels/diagnoses of schizophrenia, manic depression, bipolar disorder II, generalized anxiety disorder, etc. etc., often leave people feeling disenfranchised — no longer a part of society.

I would like to re-look at the whole issue of labels and understanding of disorders of the brain in perhaps a new light. Labels, in and of themselves, are neither good nor bad. Consider the following very real example from my own household:

"MOM!!!! Someone put your underwear in my drawer again!!!" Although my teenage daughter is several inches taller than I am and continues to grow, I alas have only gained in the width department. The underwear industry doesn't seem to care whether you are growing up or out when it comes to their size requirements. To insure unconfused undergarments, I have become "Hanes", and she's "Fruit of the Loom."

In spite of clearly marked labels on the said undergarments, the laundry helpers (those non-Hanes/non-FTL wearing members of the family) have occasional slip-ups. Labels... you'd think they would help. While this seems trivial, if you've ever put on the wrong underwear, you'd appreciate the fact that labels do come in handy.

On the far end of the spectrum, however, labels can be used to hurt and damage. Several years after the group home incident, I attended graduate school at a prestigious Mid-western university (if any of you care to listen to me sing "Hail to the Victors" I will be happy to oblige.). While in graduate school, I had the outstanding opportunity to be a teaching fellow under one of the most inspiring professors the university has ever known. Although she could have used the title of "Doctor" she preferred to simply be called "Liz". Liz had her Ph.D. in nursing and taught nursing at this university for many, many years. She had been a technical advisor for a TV show because of her decorated nursing services in Viet Nam (volunteered, not drafted). She had pioneered many patient care and teaching techniques — particularly in services for persons with chronic mental illness. Long before services for persons with chronic mental illness were ever deemed as something necessary, she was advocating for their rights and recognizing their needs. In retrospect, I realized that I learned more from working with her than I did in most of my classes.

Liz taught me the importance of accurate assessment and diagnosis of the persons we were providing services for. It was critical to get a handle on all their needs (medical, emotional, social, spiritual, and psychiatric) so that optimal health could be sought. The diagnoses, or labels if you will, allowed for a common language with all the health care providers.

Labels, alas, can also be used to separate/segregate us as I was soon to realize once again. One day, Liz invited me to join her for lunch. The waitress took my order and turned away to leave. Confused, I called her back to take the doctor's order. Very disgusted the waitress did so (The 'label' muttered NOT under her breath took my breath away.). After the waitress left, Liz sadly acknowledged that similar things happened all too frequently. You see, Liz has lived with the unthinkable label of "less than" as she is African American and I am not.

So the problems with labels come not only from the values that outside people may place on those particular labels, but also in the meanings of those labels. In 1996, my book *The Psychiatric Tower of Babble* was published. Several years later, people still ask how I came up with such a title for my book. The title was actually quite simple. Based on my years of working at the group home and then for community mental health agencies serving persons with developmental disabilities, coupled with several years of graduate school working in a long term psychiatric hospital allowed for me to develop what I consider a bilingual education. That is, I can speak the language of both disabilities and psychiatry.

The abilities to be bilingual in both developmental disabilities and psychiatry was brought home to me as not being a universal phenomena the day I worked with nursing students in the even more forgotten wards of a long-term psychiatric facility. I had long since noticed Eric on this unit and several times wondered how he had come to be here. Eric had all the classical stigmata of a person with Down syndrome or Mongoloidism as it was known at the time that he came into the state facility. He spent his days aimlessly wandering down the hallways of the institution, long since having given up hope that people would stop for any sort of conversation with him. In the word's of Yukon Cornelious, in the Christmas classic TV show, *Rudolph the Red-nosed Reindeer*, "even among misfits, he was a misfit."

My students stumbled across Eric's admitting records from 1953. The intake psychiatry report noted, "It is obvious from his facial expressions, that Eric is having difficulty dealing with his *unconscious psychic repressions* (italics mine) and will require long term psychiatric hospitalization. Prognosis: poor." Clearly, back in the days when people who were deemed different were placed in some type of long-term care facility, Eric had made it into the wrong one. By the time I came to Eric's ward, he was succumbing to the ravages of Alzheimer's Disease and it was doubtful that he would ever leave the facility to live in anything remotely resembling a normal community existence.

Discrepancies in communication took me back to the following Bible passage, and thus the title of the previous book. The Tower of Babel as written in Genesis 11:1, 5-9: "Now the whole world had one language and a common speech. . . . but the Lord came down to see the city and the tower that the men were building. The Lord said, 'If as one people speaking the same language they have begun to do this, then nothing they plan to do will be impossible for them. Come let us go down and confuse their language so they will not understand each other.' So the Lord scattered them from there all over the earth and they stopped building the city. That is why it is called Babel because there the Lord confused the language of the whole world."

As pointed out in Genesis, without a common language, joint efforts among people become impossible. Although the biblical Tower of Babel must be understood from the perspective of the people's rebellion against God, the difficulties of speaking confused languages is not uncommon — particularly in the mental health field. People in psychiatry refer to SSRI's, neurotransmitters, GABA receptors, the Cytochrome P450 System, or even unconscious psychic repressions.

People in the field of developmental disabilities, however, have THEIR own distinct language too that will include such things as behavior treatment plans, contingency plans, negative consequences, person centered planning, with many behaviors punctuated by graphs and charts. The following scenario is an all too real example of the "quandaries" when two different languages are brought into the same treatment room.

Group home and day program staff bring Jane Smith in for a psychiatric consult. Jane is diagnosed with profound mental retardation. The home has charts of 47 episodes of verbal aggression, 16 episodes of physical aggression, and 12 episodes of property disruption for the month of April. Data from the day program is quite similar. Jane has been on Mellaril 200 mg for over 15 years. The new psychiatrist looks out at the sea of faces that comprise Jane's treatment team, without a clue. The psychiatrist sees no symptoms of schizophrenia and definite signs of tardive dyskinesia (serious long-term side effect of antipsychotic medications). Worried about the tardive dyskinesia, and baffled by the graphs, the psychiatrist sends Jane and the staff home with a prescription for Mellaril 150 mg and a return appointment in three months. Staff are not given their own personal prescriptions for Valium, and consequently are even more anxious than they were prior to the appointment.

The labels, the language, and the perspectives that we each present can either bring us all together to help people like Jane or can pull us apart and the tower will never be built. It is hoped, as was true with *The Psychiatric Tower of Babble*, *Quandaries* will provide people with a common language and opportunities to provide more cohesive, appropriate psychiatric services for all the people like Jane that are caught in the rubble.

Chapter 2

If We Don't Know Where We've Been, How Will We Know When We Get There?

Psalms 119:105
Your word is a lamp to my feet and a light for my path.

Russell is a picture in contrast. He sat poised on the edge of his chair rubbing the legs of his pants frantically back and forth. He rocked slightly, but his voice never stopped its monotone, drawn out descriptions of his previous life. He couldn't look at me, but he seemed willing to tell his story. The sign outside the door stated that we sat in an office for staff serving persons with developmental disabilities, yet Russell's insight and conversations bore little resemblance to 'disabled'. He took a deep breath and started his long story.

"I can still remember the day my parents took me for a ride. They just bundled me up in clothes and said we were going out for a ride. Since I'd been kicked out of school a couple of years ago, I always enjoyed getting in the car cause it meant I would have a chance to look out and do something different. The kids used to laugh at me in my neighborhood. I'm not quite sure why. They called me "retard". I had trouble reading... I still can't read very well, but I knew I was smart, I just didn't know how to tell it. Anyway, we drove for a long, long time and then we got to "The Training School." I asked my parents where we were, and they just sat there quiet. They wouldn't tell me what this place was but I found out sure enough.

"I was sent to Cottage 17 for the new boys, but I wasn't going to get to stay there long, no sir-ee, 'cause I asked too many questions. I wanted my mom and dad to come back, but they never did. Oh, I guess about a year later they came by to see me for my birthday, but all it was, was they came and took me, we had a bite of lunch and they brought me back. I couldn't believe it! After all I told them of what was going on to me, they brought me back! After that, I guess I just didn't even care if they came to visit cause it wasn't gonna make any difference.

"I learned to run my own life, but I got in trouble with the olders. I can't sleep very well at night, even today, because back then you never knew when the olders were going to come on you. I'd be laying there in bed and if you weren't all wrapped up tight sometimes the olders could get under the covers and nobody was going to stop them. If you yelled and screamed, the staff they would just come up and make you stand there.

"Do you know what a standing is? A standing is when they bring you and make you stand with nothing to lean against and your arms up in the air and that would start about midnight and if you let your arms drop before 6:00 a.m. when the next shift came on, they beat you up, that's what a standing is. So you learned not to scream when the olders came and got you in bed, but you didn't know which was worse, being gotten in bed or the standing. I guess I still don't know today which one is worse, they both seem pretty bad to me."

Russell's story went on for over an hour and a half and I am quite certain that I only got a thumbnail's sketch of what his life was like in the institution. While Russell's story is tragically not unique, it was told more eloquently than some others have been able to share. People new to the field of disabilities are quite certain that they are not now, nor would they ever have been, as victimizing as staff /families/peers were a 'long time' ago. This same argument is heard when one deals with prejudice against African Americans:"I didn't sell any slaves, I didn't own any slaves, why am I being held responsible for the prejudices of today?" Just like my experience with Dr. Liz showed, people today still discriminate/neglect/abuse others. We must never forget that if we work for the system of mental health/disabilities, our name badge ce ments that we are members of the system and all the history before us. Nothing on that badge guarantees that we are 'safe'. In order to foster a climate of future change, we must try to understand what did go on before us.

Like Russell, many of the people I work with today, spent a significant amount of time in institutional settings. In the not so distant past, when a child with an obvious developmental disability was born, the advice given by the authorities to the parents was to "place the child in an institution." As a matter of fact, parents were encouraged to forget that their child had ever been born. At that very first group home where I worked, I met Joe (as kind and wonderful as Joe was, he wouldn't eat the soup either). With the exception of Joe, all of the people that I mention in this book have had their names changed to protect their identity. When Joe was born with Down syndrome or 'Mongoloidism', he was placed in an institution at one-week-old on the advice of the delivering physician. Distraut beyond belief, yet trusting the professionals' advise, his parents placed Joe in the State Home, and the family tried to forget him. Joe's younger brother was then named Joe to carry on the family name. I'm not sure he was ever forgotten.

Although being placed in an institution at birth was no doubt traumatic, it was probably even worse for those individuals, like Russell, whose impairment wasn't quite as obvious at birth. Perhaps this older child's impairment was not even noticed until school age when he failed kindergarten or first grade. The teacher said in kind professional tones; "this kid is an idiot." Once labeled, using the language of the time (as an imbecile, idiot or low-grade moron) schools could refuse to teach him and send him home. The family was left with two options. They could either keep their child at home with no supports being provided, or the professionals would once again recommend "send him to the institution." Sometimes, parents were not even given the choice.

Besides the initial separation, there was another catch to placing your child in the institution. It was decided that young 'retardates' had a hard time adapting to new living situations. Parents were informed that "we the professionals will take your child but" . . .and it was a big but . . . "but once you drop him off, you (the family) are to have no contact either by phone or in person for three, six, oh let's make it nine months to help him adjust."

When I have the opportunity to travel for work, I know that our children are in the capable hands of my husband. The first night, I do handsprings on my way to the hotel bed with a book after a long, uninterrupted bubble bath. When the trip lasts longer than 48 hours, however, the children get tired of the phone calls every couple of hours to make sure that they are okay.

If faced with the same limited choices of families a few decades ago, I can only imagine (in a nightmare sort of way) leaving my child, who I bonded with before birth, in an institution and not have contact with her for extended periods of time. I refuse to imagine what it would do to me and I certainly don't want to think about what it would do to her. That awful legacy has left half-healed scars, and often-open emotional wounds in the individuals and the parents that we serve today. Even people who have never been in an institution, have had segregated schools, isolated friendships, sympathetic to hostile-ranging looks from others, and other measures to insure that their difference is not accepted as a norm.

For persons with mental illness, the first sign (generally in late teen to early 20's) of psychiatric concerns often resulted in a lifetime lease at a mental institution. The stigma of mental illness was so great, that families were often frightened to have further association with the institutionalized person.

Institutionalization was not only the end result for persons with retardation or mental illness. Up until approximately 100 years ago, persons with either mental retardation, mental illness, epilepsy, physical disability, or simply the misfortune of having been born poor, were frequently placed into work houses, institutions, or other secluded facilities as these people were considered unfit for the general society. It seems that a part of human nature reacts when they perceive another to be "different". Attempts are made to place blame on the individuals themselves so as to inoculate us from inheriting this "difference".

In the early 1900's, pioneers began to explore persons within the institutional settings and thought that perhaps the root of their difficulties were from different sources.

"Different" people were evaluated as to its cause and sent to "different" facilities. This is why I questioned Eric's place in the 'wrong' institution. People with mental illness (those who believed unusual things, heard or saw unusual events) were sent to the "insane asylums" and were frequently viewed as evil, or filled with the devil. By the 1920's, however, Sigmund Freud explored the notion that (perhaps) something else was going on within the minds of insane individuals apart from Satan. He theorized that a person's illness was based on their reaction to their childhood.

I can remember learning in my basic psychiatric nursing course in the late 1970's, that the probable cause of schizophrenia was poor parenting: strong mom, weak dad, and something bizarre called double bind communication. The medications given were called major tranquilizers as compared to Valium, which was a minor tranquilizer. The idea was that the person with schizophrenia was so anxious that the anxiety caused all the symptoms. The delusions and hallucinations were "non-functional" coping strategies. Medications were supposed to ONLY be used to allow insight-oriented therapy to work. Since I never saw the insight therapy and lots of drugs dispensed, I wondered which was real—the ward or the textbook.

During that student nurse rotation at the state psychiatric hospital, I was frightened most of the time I was there. Unfortunately fear didn't count when you had paper assignments to complete. One of my assignments was Carol. At 47, Carol had been at the state hospital for more years than I had been on this earth. I was to write down a five-minute "insight" conversation. The only remotely rational conversation I could print focused on Carol's need to brush her teeth. It had been so long since she had brushed her teeth, that no one, myself included, really wanted to talk with her. Carol's needs, confusions, and fears didn't relate to anything I had learned about in class. I just hoped that if I tried hard enough, I would be able to find out that she was improperly toilet trained, cure her, and leave her with sparkling white teeth. I got a "C" on the paper, a "B" in the class, and I didn't cure her. I did finally bring her a new toothbrush from home, but it was never used by the time the semester ended. I never wanted to return.

While life in the "insane asylums" seemed to have no hope, as Russell and others point out, the state training schools (for persons with mental retardation) were less than ideal as well. There were many theories of causation, but no idea of "cures". By the 1950's, however, families of persons with developmental disabilities began objecting to sending their children to institutions. They wanted their families intact and expected the community to help. In the early 1960's, President John F. Kennedy started a new phase of "de-institutionalization". JFK's sister (Eunice) had mental retardation and their mother Rose was determined to not put her daughter in an institution. The Kennedy's, being "the Kennedy's", could create options where others had none. Perhaps because, however, the President's sister was ultimately placed in an institution and given a lobotomy (surgical removal or destruction of part of the brain) as "treatment" of aggression, the family recognized the lack of options faced by most families. Following that "surgical intervention", neither Rose's, Eunice's nor JFK's life could ever be the same.

Lobotomies can never be reversed, years of separation could not be replaced, but new choices would be made. President Kennedy signed into law the de-institutionalization of persons with retardation and mental illness. Community Mental Health (CMH) began.

People were released from institutions and new environments were created. The idea that people with disabilities could live in real homes in real communities is largely attributed to the early pioneers and early behavior therapists. The struggle, however, was just beginning. These pioneers of education for people with disabilities were those who believed that all could be taught. Behaviorists brought new technology and new expectations. They managed to prove scientifically that people with developmental disabilities could learn if somebody bothered to teach them. The literature of the time was full of stories of people with disabilities who learned astounding skills in record time just for a bit of social interaction. This radically changed the picture of "hopeless retarded souls" into a person that could think and learn. This is a very important aspect because although Kennedy signed the law for de-institutionalization of individuals with mental retardation and mental illness, people from both within the institutional settings and in the external communities thought that this was entirely impossible.

In this time of light speed change, one aspect was firmly cemented. While reformers worked to exit people from both institutional settings, it was made very clear that persons with retardation were vastly different from persons with mental illness. State and local governments often set up two completely separate systems, based on a person's "primary disability." Since mental illness was believed to be a result of improper parenting, and the internal stress brought on by thinking of one's childhood, folks with mental retardation COULD NOT be mentally ill. Remember, as a system, we took their parents; we believed them incapable of insight (this was preferred over believing their stories), and what stress in childhood? Since people with disabilities could not be mentally ill, the two systems should never cross...and they didn't.

Also in this time of change and turmoil, people were leaving the institutions, and now children with disabilities never entered in the first place. Families expected the school systems, the medical systems, etc. to provide services for these real live people.

As people moved out of the institutions, it was come as you are . . .or more aptly come as you are on drugs! While people with developmental disabilities were not allowed to have mental illnesses, people were on psychiatric medications. No one really understood how the medications worked, or why they worked, but frankly nobody cared as long as the aversive behaviors were major- tranquilized out.

Oblivious to all this history going on around me, in 1981, I graduated with my shiny new nursing diploma, and worked in a regular community hospital. It was there that I had another major self-realization; I was not a midnight worker. After eight months of looking like a questionable survivor from "Night of the Living Dead", I needed to rejoin the waking world. Since had I liked working in the group home (and I loved the guaranteed weekends off part of this new job), I became a nurse for a community agency, serving people with developmental disabilities. The term "DD" was brand new. We had a full staff of behaviorists. They were vital, because not all 'clients' (no longer called patients) were sweet and kind. More and more people were being released from institutions with a wide variety of "negative behaviors" learned in "negative settings." The behaviorists had worked miracles in the institutions, why not in the community?

The fundamental belief of behaviorism at the time it was taught to me is that man is an empty box. There are no internal drives, emotions, and personalities that are not a direct result from outside influences. Even hallucinations and suicide were explained as negative responses to negative settings.

When it came to persons with retardation, the box was less than empty. That person simply had less brain matter to learn or not learn. Dealing with negative behaviors became a vicious cycle of staff studying the person to see what the negative behavior really was, what caused it, and what maintained it. (The ABC's of behaviorism: antecedent, behavior, and consequences.) Staff then determined positive or negative reinforcers for the new, more desirable behavior. Staff would then provide the right amount of reinforcer in the right pattern and 'abra cadabra', life should be perfect. Thanks to the truly caring efforts of many staff and especially the strength of spirit of the individuals themselves, many people grew readily in their newfound worlds. When life wasn't perfect, however, (i.e., the person wasn't compliant 100% of the time) it was simply a matter of problems with the plan. We just knew that IF staff carried out the correct plan, IF we had the right reinforcer, and IF the person was positively reinforced it should all work. Plan after plan, trial after trial, time went on and yet life did not improve for some people. MI is the cause !

The wants, needs and desires of the person themselves were never considered. This was a product of the time. We knew best and therefore we didn't have to actually ask a person with the disability about their dreams . . . in fact many people didn't even believe that a person with a disability could dream. Somewhere along the line, however, the individuals themselves and the support people involved began to say "No." Plans were trashed, and people grew.

Another pivotal point came when, as in Russell's story, we had no choice but to recognize that things had gone on in the lives of people with disabilities that we frankly didn't want to look. Therapy, and even simple recognition of their human worth, went a long way towards healing. Some may find it odd that among the first advocates for understanding the mental health and psychiatric needs of a person with a disability were those who made the graphs, dispensed the tokens, and proved that people with disabilities could learn. They were also the ones to begin to suggest that these people could feel.

As a result of these understandings, the initial hard-core beliefs of behaviorism are rarely evident today. Many professionals continue to use features of behavioral intervention. Let's face it, we all like to be reinforced by pats on the back, a smile, or my personal favorite: a paycheck. Softer features have been added with the continued attempt to understand the world of antecedents, the power of reinforcers, and how cognitive behavioral management applies to people with disabilities. These important additions do attempt to address the needs and feelings of the person in question. Even more importantly, we are beginning to explore why the behavior exists in the first place and how the person can learn to have their needs met in a better and more appropriate manner. One of the most missed lessons of behaviorism (at least by me) is the idea that all behavior has meaning. I had this lesson smack me upside the head several times and by the same person.

Randy was a fourteen-year-old young man at the time that I met him. The state was investigating the care of many young people who were suffering from malnutrition (and thus dying at an alarming rate) while living in a nursing home. In addition to the malnutrition, these individuals frequently had varying degrees of cerebral palsy and often mental retardation. One of my kids...if I could have uncontracted him from his pretzel shape...would have been 5 feet tall. He moved to my unit weighing 41 lbs! At this home (and I use that term very loosely), there was generally less than one (untrained) aide for every 12 children. Since each child required 30 - 45 minutes of assistance with each meal, you do the math. Consequently, for children still healthy enough to leave the 'home' for school, the school lunch was vital for survival.

Randy was known as a head banger. Although he had spastic quadriplegic cerebral palsy, he had the ability to move his right hand from the side of his wheelchair up to his head. The harder he tried to communicate, the harder he hit his head. Because people were concerned that he might inflict further damage upon himself, he wore a hockey helmet most hours of his waking day. During lunch, the hockey helmet was removed so that the person helping him eat would have easier access to his mouth. Since Randy had a significant amount of tongue thrust, eating lunch was a time consuming activity. Time consuming or not, however, Randy clearly enjoyed eating.

The day I met Randy at school, the person helping him eat lunch stopped the shoveling procedure (Randy was anxious not to miss a bite...probably the only time in the history of the school cafeteria that children looked forward to the school lunch) to talk with me. Out of the corner of my eye I watched the following: Randy looked at his plate then he looked at his aide and nothing happened. The second time he looked at his plate, he looked at the aide, and again nothing happened. Well, after the third time, you can guess what happened. Randy started smacking his head. I watched hands go flying (both Randy's and the aide's) and the hockey helmet was quickly snapped back in place. At this point I ventured to intervene. I commented that Randy was hungry and wanted to continue eating. Comments flew at me as quickly as the arms, "Nah, he's just doing that for attention!"

As I remembered all behaviors have meaning, it didn't take rocket science to realize that Randy was trying to tell us in the only way that he knew how that he was hungry and wanted to eat. When we didn't pay attention, he activated his only communication system.

Following the initial shower and meal, the first order of business when Randy moved to my unit (area hospital space was leased until these children could be medically cleared for community placement), was to set up a communication device. Since Randy's arm could go up from the side of his wheelchair to his head, it could also go down. An extension was place on his wheelchair with a meat counter type dinger bell. We cut out pictures from various magazines, used the ever loving stickable photo albums, and put various pictures inside the photo album.

When Randy wanted something he would ding the bell, we would provide the book and he would get excited when we came to the picture of what it was he wanted. We started out simple with such things as ice cream, pudding, and Jell-O, which were a sure bet towards positive responses given Randy was a typical 14 year old adolescent with an unquenchable appetite. Time went on, and we packed away the hockey helmet.

Randy then taught me my next round of "remember all behavior has meaning". Several months after moving in, one of my staff people came running up saying that Randy was pounding on his head again. She asked whether we should get the hockey helmet off the shelf. While Randy pounded, we went from picture to picture to picture and yet nothing seemed to be what he wanted. We considered many options including restraints, diversionary tactics, and several other unmentionable options. Fortunately, when decisions are made by committee, they always take longer than the quick response of getting the helmet and putting it back on his head.

Within a half-hour, I noticed that Randy was becoming very flushed. Thinking that perhaps he was simply over excited from all the negative responses to his picture book, I still did the basic nursing thing and took his temperature. (When all else fails, get out some equipment and get some data.) Sure enough, his temperature was over 103*F. Pulling out the next piece of equipment from the nursing arsenal, I grabbed a stethoscope and listened to his lungs. Randy had the beginnings of aspiration pneumonia. Randy knew he was getting sick. Unfortunately for Randy and us, he didn't have a picture in his book that said, "Hey, stupid, I aspirated something into my lungs and I can't get it out. Can you please help me?" Antibiotics quickly took care of the problem. The hockey helmet never was needed.

Today, the number one reason I still receive referrals as a psychiatric nurse practitioner for persons with developmental disabilities is unquestionably aggression. This aggression can take many forms, either towards themselves, towards others or towards property. I can quickly assure you, however, that as in my case with Tommy and the steel-toed work boots, aggression towards others is the one that gets noticed the fastest. What I always have to remember is the lesson that both Tommy and Randy told me, all behavior no matter how unusual appearing has meaning. Our job is to try and figure it out.

Meanwhile, back to the strange and strained time of the 70's and 80's, there was an uneasy merger between psychiatry and services for folks with disabilities. The behavioral psychologist stayed busy dispensing tokens, generating volumes of programs and we took volumes of notes. These weren't just notes, they were clinical records! The psychiatry department stayed busy dispensing the major tranquilizers. Often the dosage of medicine was tied directly to the behavioral data. Unfortunately, in many people, the major tranquilizers also created other organic problems such as Tardive Dyskinesia and other health problems. Advocates then reasoned that since psychiatric illness was impossible in persons with disabilities, then all psychiatric medicines should be abandoned. Systems all over the country tried to abolish Mellaril and Thorazine and other antipsychotics as abruptly as possible. This was disastrous for reasons that we now understand but not then. People abruptly stopped from their medications often go through a rebound phenomenon and display this horrifically uncomfortable sensation as aggression. This would then re-justify the use of Vitamin M/H, often at even higher dosages to regain "control". And so, the use of the psychotropic medications both appropriate and inappropriate continues even today.

As the cry for appropriate mental health services for persons with disabilities became heard, systems began exploring ways to adequately assess, diagnose and treat without chemically straight-jacketing people. Pioneers in the field such as Dr. Robert Sovner, Dr. Menoloscino, Dr. Fletcher, and others began writing of the co-existence of developmental disabilities and psychiatric impairment, and the field of dual diagnosis (DD/MI) grew.

Chapter 3

All Stressed Up & Nowhere to Go

Proverbs 14:30a:
"A heart at peace, gives life to the body."

RRIINNGG! "The S.A.D. Agency" (Sue's Aggression Detective Agency). When my phone rings at work, I can generally predict the reason. Someone I know is out of medications and needs a refill, someone I know is in crisis, or someone I'm about to know is in crisis. Random calls from a tele marketer are almost a relief.

Stress from most sources can cause irritability. Although I'm sure my family will vouch for my near saintly presentation when ill with the flu (at least if they still want groceries in the house, they will), not everyone is so friendly. Indeed, in my line of work, many of the people I meet in crisis (read = HHEELLPP!!, not the Chinese for 'opportunity') are aggressive. They are hurting others, hurting themselves, or practicing for their next job as a demolition worker. The support people looking for my help want instant relief for the said individual and for themselves. At times, I suspect that if I recommended continuous anesthesia, no one would object.

Before hooking up the anesthesia, however, the first step is to try to gather enough information to make a remote guess at what is happening. Unlike green nasal gunk that generally means a sinus infection, aggression is a very nonspecific behavior that means something. Randy's aggression (head banging) meant anything from "I'm hungry" to "I have crud in my lunges." Aggression can result from countless combinations of reasons. Even within the same person, the same external behavior (i.e., throwing furniture out the window) could relay numerous internal problems.

When I first began working for my present employer, I was baffled much of the time even with my bilingual education. I remember sitting down at a psychiatry appointment for a consumer and hearing: "Fred had 3.4 acts of aggression in May, 5.7 acts of aggression in June, and by July, he had 12.5 acts of aggression!" I spent much of the meeting trying to figure out what ".7" act of aggression was. The doctor (who didn't know either) couldn't see any signs of psychosis, and so LOWERED the Haldol (prompting staff to reconsider their need for employment!). Unfortunately, counts /averages/ estimates of aggression mean very little when it comes to diagnosing mental illness. While aggression should never be ignored, it should also never be considered the diagnostic endpoint.

Let's consider the errors that can occur if one only looks at the numbers or averages of aggressive acts. Suppose that every time I walk past the secretary in the next cube, I tap her on the shoulder. The behavior treatment specialist (whose cube is across from ours) could dutifully record these episodes on a chart, figure out the numbers of days I was in the office for the month, and come up with an average of 29.7 tapping episodes (I was to eventually find out that averages give you the ".7") per workday. While highly tolerant of my horrible penmanship, talking too loud on the phone when the kids call (for the 5th time that morning), and my radio, the tapping finally gets to her. For months she has been the model of patience and understanding. One hot summer day, however, she's had it. She hides an automatic weapon in her purse and does me in at my next swipe. As this was her only act of aggression for the 3-MONTH period, her quarterly average would only be 0.017...much lower than my 29.7 daily rate and thus hers would be hardly worth mentioning! This absurd illustration proves the point that aggression, per se, must be qualified, and described by all. Numbers alone are entirely inadequate, as the aggression must also be understood in context.

For the sake of argument, let's define irritability and aggression (in a non-criminal sense) as a response to stress. Many of us can relate to acting angrily towards others when we were upset with something else. This is not simply an event that occurs to "them" (others with disabilities or mental illness), but most people. What sorts of things stress you out? Have you ever been stressed out at work because you felt you had all kinds of responsibilities but no authority to make change? Do you ever feel angry when you walk in the door from a busy day at work and are informed that you need to clean the house, cut the grass and oh, yeah, the laundry needs doing? Does fear of violence ever affect you? How about concerns of whether you have enough funds to go out for some fun or for future needs? Do family members ever let you down? Have you ever felt like you were in a dead-end job with no chance of advancement? Have you ever lost a friend for reasons that you didn't understand? Does physical illness affect you or someone you love? Now if you say these examples or more of your own never stresses you, I can only conclude one of two things: you're already comatose from reading this book, or lying.

For persons with developmental disabilities, the whole picture of being 'stressed out' takes on a whole new dimension. Various persons with disabilities relayed all these common psychological stressors listed above. Surprised? I'm sure you were led to believe that these things only affect 'us'.

Stress is any internal or external event that forces the body to adapt/respond to the given situation. Even positive events can be very stressful. When the human body perceives stress, many chemicals such as adrenaline, cortisol, and those needed for glucose (sugar) control all get in the act. People respond to stressful situations in a variety of ways. Some people display extreme emotions. Some people withdraw into themselves. Some people have trouble concentrating. Some experience physical symptoms. Many people become irritable and possibly even aggressive. These responses are not dependent on IQ, but rather on the personality and coping strategies of the individual. When stress of some sort has created enough distress to bring the individual to the attention of health care staff, it always warrants attention. The type of attention needed is only the beginning of the puzzle.

The most common cause of stress-induced aggression that I note in persons with disabilities is physical illness. Like Randy, most people, classified disabled or not, become more irritable when they feel sick. My poor husband had the misfortune of getting the flu in the middle of the summer. His head, throat, and body all ached. His temperature was around 102*F. As a nap for him seemed indicated, I left for the grocery store. I promised to pick him up a super-sized milk shake on my way home. His response: "I don't want a @#$% milkshake, I'm not hungry." Knowing this was not his usual self talking, I left Grumpy to sleep. An hour later as I walked in the door, you can guess his first comment. "Where's my milkshake?" It was strawberry.

Probably the most essential activity to occur **before** an initial psychiatric consultation is an evaluation for probable physical pain/illness. Over the recent Christmas holidays, I received a phone call that Sarah (a well-known consumer of our clinic) had had a dramatic rise in "target symptoms" (aka aggression) over the past 2 days. Given that I was walking out the door in 5 minutes for the same said holidays, I ordered labs and left. As is the tragic case in large bureaucracies, the labs were done at a different lab than usual, and our office never got them until much later. Fortunately Sarah's staff persisted during the holiday, and before I ever got the labs, her primary care doctor treated her for a urinary tract infection. In spite of the mix-ups, if we had only increased her medications for her Bipolar disorder, she could have had serious side effects, not to mention an untreated UTI. Both initially and whenever there is a worsening of target issues; a complete evaluation of physical concerns must be done to rule out any possible connection.

Common physical concerns may include seizure disorders, headaches, hypothyroidism, and gastrointestinal (GI) disturbances, such as gastric reflux, ulcers, milk intolerance, constipation, and/or diarrhea, and medication side effects.

Many of you reading this book have some medication that you will never take. Perhaps aspirin upsets your stomach. Cold preparations may make you jittery or sleepy depending on the type. Some antibiotics may give you diarrhea. Although these reactions are not allergies, *per se,* they still cause significant distress such that you will not take them. How many of the people we work with may experience intolerable side effects, but are still given the medicine by caring yet unsuspecting support people?

When it comes to physical health needs, my newest soapbox is about "that oxygen to the brain stuff." It is basic knowledge that in order for the brain to function well, it must have adequate supplies of oxygen. Sometimes, however, this most basic of information gets forgotten. Everyone assumed that 67-year old Jane's bipolar disorder had worsened. She was irritable, not sleeping well, and often appeared confused. A routine EKG at her physical, however, showed a not so routine heart block that warranted surgery. When her heart could again supply an adequate blood supply to the brain, her other symptoms resolved. Indeed, had her medication for mania been substantially increased, it could have had severe negative effects.

Brad has Down syndrome. At age 46, he had all the symptoms of Alzheimer's type dementia. An observant midnight staff worker noted that he also snored very loud then was silent for brief periods all night long. He was evaluated for sleep apnea. The use of a CPAP machine has resolved his sleep apnea. Because he is no longer deprived of oxygen each night and sleeps better, he is no longer confused, dazed, or irritable.

Rhonda has depression. In spite of increasing the dosage of her antidepressant, she remained listless, irritable, and chronically tired. Her annual labs were ordered one month early. She had severe anemia. (Severe anemia means that there are diminished red blood cells to carry oxygen to the brain, or anywhere else for that matter.) I could have doubled her Prozac dosage, but until she had enough red blood cells to carry a sufficient amount of oxygen, her depressive type symptoms were not going to clear up.

Since not all persons with disabilities can independently list their symptoms, investigative diagnostic work is usually necessary. This too is true for most people, but may be more complex here. In the days of mangled, er, managed care, it is often difficult to justify the more expensive tests. MRI's are not necessary for all people. When Cheryl was so aggressive that she required 2:1 staffing even after multiple drug trials, more extensive health testing was suggested. Ultimately, the MRI of the brain showed a small but growing tumor. Surgery, NOT, Haldol was the answer. In cases such as these, the testing is expensive, but nothing else could have helped. When the assessment process starts, basic laboratory screenings should include, blood counts, liver and kidney function tests, thyroid screens, urinalysis, and others based on the individual needs of the person. I have also had uncommon success with finding positive results for the *h.pylori* bacteria that causes GERD and ulcers. It also goes without saying that a primary health provider who has an interest in the person and is willing to use nonverbal assessment cues for evaluation is an essential luxury.

Jack rolled his wheelchair into the conference room; he was a pleasant man who seemed well liked by all that knew him. He had lived in a nursing home for over thirty years because of his cerebral palsy and 'chronic psychotic disorder.' Due to federal guidelines, a screening process brought him to the attention of the community mental health staff. After a bit of time and a lot of preparation, he moved. He loved his new group home, new friends, and particularly his new girlfriend.

Although the community doctor continued his 20-year history of Mellaril 200 mg at bedtime, people were concerned that the medication was no longer working. He was becoming 'more psychotic.' Perhaps the stress of the move was too much for him. He had lost 20 pounds, which was a concern, as he was quite thin to begin with. What really scared the staff, however, was his insistence that the 'wolves were howling at his door', and many nonspecific physical complaints of discomfort.

At first glance, Jack may have been psychotic, but some things did not fit. Most people with any type of schizophrenia (especially if the condition is worsening) have extreme difficulty with social situations. Jack loved to be with people, and people enjoyed being with him. He looked to me like someone who simply didn't feel well (How's that for a succinct diagnosis?). He was due to see his primary care doctor again soon. We all agreed that close attention should be given to the weight loss and discomfort.

Jack had cancer. Other seniors from his former nursing home had often referred to dying as 'the wolves howling at the door.' Jack was not then, and possibly never was psychotic. Given the type of cancer that he had, it is doubtful that even earlier intervention could have helped. What is important is to never overlook what a person is saying (verbally or non-verbally) and when we don't think that what they say makes sense, perhaps finding an explanation might be in order!

Although not classified as illnesses, practitioners should always be on the lookout for potential genetic syndromes. Specific syndromes are often associated with common physical or psychiatric issues. For example, persons with Down syndrome have many common health concerns. Heart defects, spinal column defects (which must be assessed before any physical exercise program is begun or paralysis or even death could result), and sinus problems are not uncommon. By age 25, all persons with Down syndrome should have annual thyroid studies. The prevalence rates of hypothyroidism are over 30%! In psychiatry, we know that autistic features, depression, and Alzheimer's type dementia can occur with alarming frequency. Other common syndromes with physical and/ or psychiatric concerns include Fragile X, Prader Willi, PKU, Lesch-Nyhan, Autism Spectrum disorders, and fetal alcohol exposure.

Once we get past the physical concerns, we must then consider psychological/social stresses. Psychological stress can come from both inside our self and from our relationship with the outside world. People with a developmental disability often suffer from many social crises. They suffer from the stigma of being disabled and are frequently looked down upon by others within a society that worships the ideal. In years past (and even today, if we are being honest with ourselves), they have been treated with many degrading approaches such as institutionalization, infantilization, and a requirement to be compliant.

Are you ever non-compliant? Please don't stand up and be counted, the number would be past what my calculator could reasonably expect to manage. Forced compliance is a source of major stress – for anyone. I remember a shopping trip with a distant relative. This particular lady is well accustomed to being in charge of both herself and others around her. She's one of those people who is always impeccably groomed and in the latest of fashion. I, on the other hand, am grateful that blue jeans and cotton knit shirts, (long or short sleeve depending on the weather) are never entirely in or out of style.

On this particular shopping trip, I spotted a beautiful suit marked seventy-five percent off!! If there's one thing I love more than comfortable clothes, it's a bargain. Alas, the suit was made of wool and just touching it caused my skin to break out in an allergic rash. I put it back. My companion/relation noticed me putting back what was probably the only potential wardrobe item she'd ever approved of. She commented, "You really dress too casual." She paused, and then continued "And you're not going to change because I've spoken are you?" I'm not. I'm definitely a 'non-compliant' kind of person. While I didn't back down, thinking of that situation still raises my blood pressure several notches.

While at a speaking engagement, a very concerned staff person approached me. He wanted to know if there was some anti-anxiety medicine that would help his consumer relax during her haircut. She screamed and yelled and hit others whenever it was time for a haircut. Clearly she was non-compliant and aggressive as well. As we discussed the situation, it was noted that this non-verbal person was virtually never aggressive except at haircut time. We concluded that perhaps rather than a medication, letting her 'choose' to wear her hair long, made more sense. She was being forced to comply with something she didn't like. Her only alternative was to strike out.

Although this book is unable to devote a lot of space to the area of abuse, it is an area that requires a lot of emphasis. As a cause of psychological stress, abuse is a reality all too frequently. This abuse may not be current in action, but very current in memory. We often discover anniversary dates (of the trauma), people who look, act, sound, or even smell like the abuser, or recent contact with the abuser to start the avalanche of memories and thus crisis. The abuse that persons with developmental disabilities have endured at the hands of the very people hired to help them is nothing less than an abomination. There are many excellent resources (Hingsburger; Ryan; Sobsey) regarding the nature and response of physical and/or sexual abuse in persons with disabilities. It goes without saying, however, that a population of people

where huge numbers have been abused will endure –
perhaps forever – the stress of living in environments
where they were hurt, surrounded by people they no
longer feel they can trust.

Yes, stress is a universal phenomenon, not just for persons with disabilities. When you are faced with stress,
what do you do? Eat more? Sleep more? Talk to other
people? Do you scream and yell? Now, if a person with
a developmental disability screams and yells, that person
is subject to a behavior treatment plan. We run away to
the mall. They 'elope'. We go to the bar and have a drink.
They are not allowed to engage in unhealthy life choices.
We eat an extra bowl of double chocolate ice cream, they
find the refrigerator locked.

I remember the day I got so angry with my husband (about
what, I no longer remember) that I left him with the children while I went shopping. Walking through the mall
calmly looking at all the things I couldn't afford soothed
me almost as much as being alone without husband and
kids in tow. Oh, I know what I did was 'unhealthy.' I
knew I would send hundreds of self-help writers running to their computers. I knew that I had to deal with
the original problem plus his anger at my unexplained
leaving, but I also knew that I HAD to get out of there.
Where I am different from a person with a disability who
elopes from a stressful environment is that I had no treatment plan to face when I returned.

My best friend, unfortunately, lives another telephone area code away. Our phone bills are usually in the three digits. We have solved many of the world's crises (at least within our worlds) on the telephone. Next to our mates, we have been each other's primary source of support. Many people with disabilities do not have somebody that they can call on the telephone who is not a relative or a paid staff. There is no one that they can just 'kavetch' to about what is going on in their lives. Even if they did, they would have to wait until it is 'their night to make a phone call.'

I don't know if you have ever read the 'DD Handbook.' This is not a published book, but a hidden set of rules found in almost every agency. According to most "DD Handbooks", if you are developmentally disabled, you cannot exceed your ideal body weight by more than ten percent. It's a rule. One of many found in The Book. If you do go over ten percent of your ideal body weight, you can kiss the double chocolate ice cream goodbye. On Christmas Eve when everyone else is having a feast, you are going to eat carrot sticks because treatment plans know no season.

I am not diagnosed as having a disability but someone could look at me and say, "Sue, you need to lose twenty pounds" (and that's if they're being kind). And guess what they would find if they investigated a little further? My father had two heart attacks. My mother also has a heart condition. WAIT! My brother has high blood pressure. Now, I'm a reasonably intelligent sort of a person. I can figure out what the odds are against me, but it's still my choice. The correct behavior treatment plan has yet to be written to change my occasional stops into McDonald's.

I had just started to see clients on my own. Reading through the doctor's notes, I saw that Bill was basically stable. Whew! I can handle this. I called Bill and his team into the meeting room. I was immediately informed of Bill's aggression level, which had gone through the roof. He was stealing food, was non-compliant (particularly to the rule about staying out of the kitchen), and would elope to the local food store. So much for the doc's only giving me stable clients.

It turns out that shortly after his last psychiatric visit, Bill had his annual planning meeting. Middle age spread to the tune of 25.2 lbs over ideal body weight was identified, quantified, and planned for reversal. He was placed on a twelve hundred-calorie diet. His 'negative' behaviors made sense to me – he was reacting to forced compliance. The stress of living with people who felt they could just do this to him was too great for him. He was angry. The true irony of the situation was that Bill and I were the thinnest people in the room!

Developmentally delayed? We, the experts, coined the term 'developmentally delayed'. This implies that some people require a longer time to develop. Maybe this 'delay' requires attention. Please do not interpret my line of thinking as the same as seeing a person with a disability as an 'eternal child'. What I am implying is that persons with disabilities may not have had adequate opportunities to learn coping strategies to handle their stresses. (Trust me, though, not many of my coping strategies are grown-up either.) True mental health is the ability to enjoy life, and cope with difficulties as they come in a reasonable fashion. While this is true regardless of intellectual functioning, the conflict between coping strategies available and types of stresses may become even greater the older the person becomes. In adulthood the stress of choosing between jobs or between possible living situations are greater than those involved in the choices we made as children. It is important that coping strategies grow along with the demands made.

Jessie at age 34 was experiencing some major stressors when I first met her. She had the desire and skills to work and live more independently. Unfortunately, when challenged by stress, she reverted into what would be typical teenage rebellion (her maturational age = 13-14 years old). Teenagers are at an age where they still require adult guidance and structure, but in developing their own identity they also try to break away and defy those supports.

After Jessie finished crying the very first day we met, I made a brilliant observation, "You look sad." She agreed. I followed that observation with a remarkable question, "Why?" She told me. Jessie's major concern was whether she could in fact continue to support herself once out of the group home. A friend of hers had 'acted bad' (had a psychotic decompensation) and was returned to the institution. She said that while she hated the institution, she knew she would always 'have a roof over my head and three meals a day.' Acting bad in order to return to the institution equaled safety for her. She understood the possible consequences of a move to a new apartment. "If I screw up in my own apartment, I could end up a bag lady on the street." Her aggressions and swearing must be seen as 'typical' or understandable for a 14-year-old, but she has never learned how a 34-year old handled the stress of her first apartment.

There are certainly positive ways to deal with stress: talking with others, hugs, taking a nap, even planned elopements. Many people can feel better by going for a walk or most any sort of exercise. Much as I hated to admit it, when I realized I was taking no less than 3 different medications for stomach upset, I had to do something. "Something" meant starting to exercise regularly for the first time in my life. While I am still overweight, I am actually more physically fit per a cardiac stress test than I was when I was thinner. Some people feel better after listening to choice music. Faith life can be very relaxing. In fact, some studies have noted that those people with a deep faith life typically live longer, healthier lives – even with the usual amounts of problems.

Andrew arrives to our church each Sunday that he can with the most beautiful smile. I do not know of anyone who loves to be there more. He greets others enthusiastically, sings joyfully, and listens with his heart. Since Andrew lives in a group home 50 miles from the church, his church attendance is sporadic. One visit coincided with a Sunday when Holy Communion was not being served. His tears prompted the elders to rapidly prepare communion for all. Since Andrew has Down syndrome, his understanding of communion on "first and third Sundays of the month only" exceeded his understanding of time **and** church rules. Watching his joy allowed us all to receive extra peace on the fourth Sunday.

For some people, excessive stressors and often-inadequate stress relievers, however, (there are only so many donut holes and diet Pepsi's that any one person can use for consolation) can tip the balance towards aggression and even mental health concerns. The human body is an incredible collection of intimately-intertwined parts. No one system performs without affecting other portions of the body. This is why a stomachache can reduce your ability to function at work. The question becomes what happens when severe stress effects a minimally functioning portion of the body?

I have a weakened GI system in part due to milk intolerance. If I have milk, my immediate environment is distinctly unfriendly. When I am faced with some sort of crisis, my weakened system is quickly affected. I have diarrhea or stomach upset. These pressing needs make it difficult to deal with anything else in my world. I stop being a competent adult, an effective decision-maker, and my skills as a communicator deteriorate until I'm left with only two sentences – Get out of my way! And Get out of the bathroom –NOW! This isn't really a moral weakness; I was born with a 'defect' in how my body operates.

Using this same analogy, it goes without saying that individuals with a developmental disability generally have an inherent defect somewhere within the brain. This defect may have been a result of damage *in utero,* at the time of birth, or shortly after birth, but for some reason, the brain did not develop, as it should have. This provides a 'weakness' in the system such that other pathologies can occur. It comes as no surprise that seizure disorders are far more common in people with a developmental disability.

Brain changes, biochemical stresses, social stresses, abuses, and limited supports do not add up to a mentally healthy individual. For all of these reasons, eventually, it was conceded that not only could persons with developmental disability have psychiatric dysfunctions, but also they were more likely than the average person to have a psychiatric problem. Some estimates state the numbers may be as high as thirty to thirty-five percent of all persons with developmental disabilities may have an additional psychiatric impairment.

If you are willing to agree that persons with developmental disabilities can have a mental illness, what does that mean? Are drugs always necessary? Mental illness is a physical illness. While a person's happiness and well-being can be affected by good and bad situations in life, mental illness has a definite physiological basis. So what's the difference between treatment of mental health, mental illness and chemical restraint?

I am not an advocate of medications in all cases. I do not receive a 'kickback' for the amount of medicines prescribed. I understand that in the past, persons with mental retardation were either over-medicated (we've all seen dazed, drugged eyes) or horribly under-medicated. People with disabilities were often routinely operated on without anesthesia! I doubt anyone reading this book today would deny any one, regardless of IQ status, the right to have anesthesia during surgery. If psychiatric medications help persons with so-called normal intelligence, should they not also be available to persons with developmental disabilities? If you answer yes, then the next question is in what cases should they be prescribed?

Have you ever had a really bad cold or flu? You feel downright awful. My mom always called it feeling "Aus gescheissen" (if you're German you'll understand why I didn't translate that!). If you don't go to the doctor, it will take about four to seven days to feel better. If you do go to the doctor, you expect some magical cure. Sometimes the patient feels so bad, they insist on a prescription for antibiotics. You will still feel better in four to seven days. Antibiotics do absolutely nothing for viruses that cause the common cold and flu. In fact, improper overuse of antibiotics has led to the creation of 'super bugs', bacteria that are very resistive to our current supply of antibiotics. The person is also at risk for side effects of the antibiotics. Antibiotics, however, may help avoid or cure a secondary opportunistic bacterial infection. When a person is in a weakened condition from a cold or flu virus, bacteria can move in and cause their own infection. Some people may swear that antibiotics are helping, but this is simply the 'placebo' effect (we feel better because we really *think* it helps, not because it does help).

Medicines used in psychiatry can have much the same effect. In many instances, a person has been placed on the 'drug of the month' hoping and praying that it helps curb negative behaviors, typically aggression and 'noncompliance'. If the person has no actual psychiatric illness, the medicine will have no effect (other than the initial placebo) at best to harmful side effects at worst. This is chemical restraint and should be avoided at all costs. On the other hand, if actual psychiatric illness does exist, it requires accurate assessment, diagnosis and treatment that may very well include *appropriate* medications in amounts that create the maximum amount of benefit with the least number of side effects.

The next few chapters will discuss the primary psychiatry categories, and their association in persons with disabilities.

Chapter 4

Depression: Life In The Pits

Psalms 6:3
My soul is in anguish. How long, o lord, how long?

Since I don't drink coffee, and diet Pepsi comes in its own convenient container, my husband is the primary bene-factor of the gift mugs bearing the names of various psy-chiatric drugs brought to my office by pharmaceutical vendors. I know that by using these coffee mugs, he pro-vides free advertising for the products. On the other hand, given the frequency with which he has misplaced them, or put them on the hood of the car and then driven off, it seems better to provide free advertising than to go out and buy new coffee mugs all the time. Did you know that a Prozac coffee mug could withstand flying off a car going in reverse at approximately 20 miles an hour, bounc-ing onto a dirt road and still remain intact? Alas, the cof-fee did spill out. I like the mug for its durability factor;

Charlie says he likes the Prozac mug because it's a name that people recognize. Many of the other mugs have names on them that most people couldn't pronounce, much less recognize.

In 1999, three of the top 25 medications prescribed in the United States were antidepressants. I'm not sure if the rate of depression has risen that fast, recognition of depression has increased, or if medication is seen as the fast way to feeling better from many of the common ailments prevalent in our society. The most recent statistics indicate that depression is one of the most expensive conditions in the US both in terms of lost productivity and actual treatment costs. While these numbers are impressive, we must never forget the individuals with depression and their suffering. This illness devastates not only the individual's life, but also the life of those around him or her.

Diane was reminded of her appointment with me for a recheck of her antidepressant medications at the last possible second. She came rushing into the appointment from spring-cleaning her apartment with a smile on her face and the most disheveled sweat suit I had seen in quite some time. In spite of the less than vogue outfit, she had the beauty and regal bearing of an exotic princess. This is in stark contrast to when we first met. When I first evaluated Diane three or four years ago, her mother brought her into the community mental health building. She shuffled as she walked. She almost ran into a wall because she was looking down at the floor as opposed to where she was going. Although her outfit that day was equally disheveled, the pronounced body odor, poor eye contact, and the very soulful expression on her face were dead giveaways that something was amiss.

Her mother explained (because Diane was almost unable to speak) that over the past three to six months, Diane had dropped out of all of her familiar and favorite activities. She lost her job at a local department store when she phoned in sick too many times. The soprano section of her church choir sorely missed her since she hadn't shown up for practice in several months. Diane lost 19 pounds in 3 months because she simply didn't have the desire to eat. She was attempting to sleep 20 out of 24 hours a day and still complained of being tired. When she was awake, her face was tear-streaked. What few words I could pull out of her consisted of "God wishes that I were dead and sometimes I wish I was dead too".

Although Diane was also diagnosed with mild mental retardation, her symptoms had nothing to do with her intellectual functioning and everything to do with the biochemical disturbances in her brain.

According to the late, great Dr. Sovner, persons with developmental disabilities suffer from the full range of psychiatric disorders. Unfortunately, these disorders often present as "negative behaviors". If after ruling out medical, environmental, and other reasons for the negative behavior (often aggression), we must consider psychiatric concerns. The most prevalent of the psychiatric illnesses in persons with developmental disabilities are the Affective Disorders, or mood disorders as they are oftentimes called. The affective disorders include depression and manic depression (bipolar disorder).

According to the sales of antidepressants, most people reading this book probably know of someone who has been diagnosed with major depression. If you do know somebody with untreated major depression, stop and think about what it is like interacting with that individual. Depressed people can pull your own mood down. If the person does talk, it is almost always of a negative subject or mood. Nothing is ever fun, good, or happy. You may hear themes of "I'm sorry "or "I'm bad." Their self-care is the pits.

When I work with people who are clinically, chronically depressed, frankly I sometimes feel the desire to smack them upside the head. (Fortunately I don't have somebody with a chart - at least that I am aware of - counting all of my desires for acts of aggression if not actual attempts.) No, I am not suggesting that all clinicians go out and smack their consumers upside the head, but I suspect anger is one reaction that you might have when associating with somebody with depression.

Consider the following conversation, husband to wife, "Heather, if you just got yourself into the shower. If you just put on a little make up. If you just came with the kids and me to the restaurant you would start to feel better, honest you would." After a long lengthy pause,

Heather glances over George's way and mutters, "Nothing will ever be any good again. Don't you understand? I can't get out of the house. I can't make myself move. Nothing will ever feel right again. You guys just leave without me. I am better off dead." George's inclination to shake some sense into Heather is understandable, but it won't fix the problem.

I am equally sure you know somebody who requires insulin for diabetes. Diabetes is an illness where the pancreas (located somewhere on the middle to left-hand side of your belly) is no longer producing enough insulin. When you eat, insulin is necessary to move the sugar found in most foods out of your blood stream and into the body's cells to be used as energy. Without insulin, the person with Type I Diabetes could eat daily super-sized meals, but within days to weeks he will feel ill and could even die of cell starvation. Although people with diabetes also have to watch their diet, take care of their skin, watch their eyes, and exercise, without insulin the person will eventually die.

In my best clinical judgment, (and even the "Inquirer" hasn't said so), I can pretty much assume that punching the individual with diabetes in the stomach will NOT get the pancreas producing the appropriate amount of insulin. The bottom line at this time is the person with insulin dependent diabetes requires shots on an at least once-a-day basis. (As a note to my friend the diabetic educator, see I was paying attention!) Back to George and Heather:

Heather's brain cells are experiencing their own form of starvation –brain chemical starvation.

The brain is the central processing unit for the entire human body. My sister-in-law has an expression that her children know well, "If Mama ain't happy, ain't nobody happy." Like many moms, she is her family's central organizing unit; she keeps up with everyone's schedules, needs, jobs, etc. When she is exhausted, sick, or simply out of sorts, "ain't nobody happy."

Working as our body's CPU, our brains' functions are vital and varied. It's responsible for maintaining memories from our senses, experiences and educational opportunities. Memory comes in many forms. It is divided into immediate recall, past recall and remote recall. If any of you really care, I can still recall all four verses to "My Love is Like a Red, Red Rose" that I learned in fifth grade (very, very remote recall). Past recall allows you to smell cinnamon and remember Grandma's cookies. Immediate recall allows us to look at a phone number and remember it long enough to dial the phone. Most of us, however, unless we store the number in long-term memory, will not recall it 5 minutes later. This last example is actually referred to as 'working memory.' The brain also takes in all the information that I gather from my senses (see, taste, smell, touch and hear), and helps me to act on it. For example, when I see smoke coming from the toaster, hear the smoke alarm, and smell the charcoaled bread, I respond by popping up the toast, turning off the alarm and yelling, "Charlie, your toast is done!"

Our brains monitor our abilities to solve problems and plan for the future. For example, do I want to use a double coupon now for this box of cereal or hope that the store has this cereal on sale next week to use with my double coupon? I must also call on my memory to remember if anyone in the household even likes this kind of cereal. Since I like to complete a weekly shopping trip in less than 2 hours, this is all done very quickly. Other parts of our brain help regulate mobility, maintain balance, and assist our athletic prowess. Additionally, brains are also responsible for our moods, intellect, artistic talents, many hormonal activities, and so many more functions that it almost defies understanding.

While scientists can write a basic job description for the brain, it is still considered by many to be the last great frontier. Scientists worldwide are trying to determine how the brain is formed, what areas are responsible for which brain actions, and how these sections communicate with one another. Sometimes, even though a section of brain may die i.e., after a stroke, other portions of the brain may actually take over such that the person restores some, if not all, function. What is ironic about the highly complex nature of the brain is that in the brain, brain cells don't actually touch one another.

If one could get a microscope small enough to take a close look at the nerve cells (Chart 4.1), you would be amazed at the lack of physical connections. Although neurons (nerve cells and neurons mean the same thing) are often specialized and structured in pathways in the brain, they

Neurotransmission Illustration

(Chart 4.1)

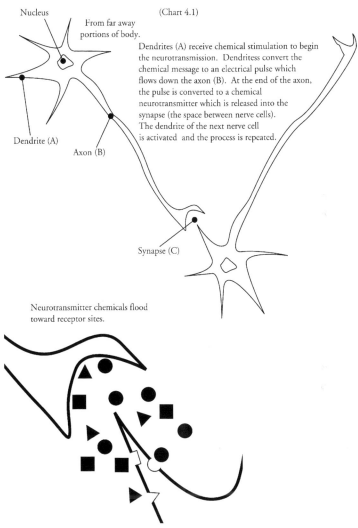

Nucleus

From far away
portions of body.

Dendrites (A) receive chemical stimulation to begin
the neurotransmission. Dendritess convert the
chemical message to an electrical pulse which
flows down the axon (B). At the end of the axon,
the pulse is converted to a chemical
neurotransmitter which is released into the
synapse (the space between nerve cells).
The dendrite of the next nerve cell
is activated and the process is repeated.

Dendrite (A)

Axon (B)

Synapse (C)

Neurotransmitter chemicals flood
toward receptor sites.

communicate with one another with chemicals called neurotransmitters (or neurochemicals) as opposed to touching each other. These neurotransmitters transmit information from one nerve cell to another. When there is a screw-up in the chemical transmission system of the brain, such as too much or too little of the neurotransmitter going from one nerve cell to the other, mental illness occurs. That's right, mental illness is NOT a result of poor toilet training etc., but rather a chemical imbalance in the brain.

I am not an Internet expert. In fact, I am limited to scanning a few sites programmed by others, and checking the e-mail (most of which are for our daughter). What little I have learned, however, is the importance of the correct "address". Failing to put a little "." in, or missing one letter can send your original search into cyberspace. I am told that there is a lot of information in cyberspace, but care must be taken in trying to find it. While the keys of a keyboard (what do people who don't use our alphabet do?) direct cyberspace, the information to and from our brains is just as finely tuned and directed by the neurochemicals.

Information in psychiatry is rapidly evolving. By the time this book is finished, some researcher will hopefully find another piece to the complex puzzle. When medicines like Prozac first came on the market, we had a simple explanation of depression being a serotonin deficiency (hence, Heather's 'brain starvation'). It ain't so simple any more. We have come to understand that for any given brain disorder, there is generally more than one neurotransmitter involved. In addition, problems in the chemical system can occur both within and outside the brain cells. Brain cells are ever changing. Cells add and prune off connections to other brain cells continuously. It truly is the case of "use it or lose it". Brain cells like to be exercised by a variety of stimuli. By the way, too much TV is thought to decrease brain connections. If I were a social climber (women who like to can their own garden produce, hang clothes on the clothes line even in November, and live in blue jeans are not exactly on the social ladder of success!), it would be all about connections. In terms of brainpower, it is still about connections.

Problems may also arise because of actual structural changes in the brain such as too large fluid spaces, or too small of a particular section. Unfortunately, our abilities to assess and evaluate actual brains remain very limited, even with the new technology. In the future, as experience and research will show, however, to the extent that we can better understand these effects, we will be better able to diagnose problems, and even more importantly, treat them.

As discussed in the previous chapter about stress, there are many reasons to suppose that an individual with a developmental disability and in particular mental retardation would have a higher than average risk of a psychiatric impairment. These include the atrocious histories of abuse, the frequently untaught or at least unlearned coping strategies, and the higher than average stress that these individuals face. Compound this with difficulties in communication and it is understandable why psychological stress would occur. In a brain with structural abnormalities (as would be expected in a person with a brain related disability), it should be no surprise then, that the concentration of neurotransmitters and receptor sites in those areas might also be out of whack. While this might explain the higher rates of psychiatric impairment in persons with developmental disabilities, we must still consider the many difficulties in terms of assessment, diagnosis and particularly treatment.

1. Since the global diagnosis of mental retardation can arise from any number of reasons, the potential structural concerns will also vary. Very rarely is the cause of mental retardation listed in the files available by the time someone is 36 years of age and first reaches the psychiatric intake desk. On occasion, time permits for an extensive review of the records (I blast right past the 3 inches of progress notes on the toothbrushing program), and once in a great while, the historical notes will give a clue as to the cause of the disability. That, or having someone who knew them "when" may give us a clue. More often than not, however, the information is simply unknown.

2. Neurological imaging such as an MRI, or CT Scan, may elicit the structural malformations of the brain, but these tests are very expensive and mangled, er, managed care programs rarely will pay for them. In spite of this, once done, practitioners can gain

valuable information. Consider the case of the individual with microcephaly. Darrin is a 28 year-old young man who truly fulfills the criteria for attention deficit hyperactivity disorder (ADHD). While evaluating his seizures, a CT Scan noted that Darrin has almost no frontal lobe. To those in the know on ADHD, the frontal lobe is responsible for attention span, impulse control, and a lot of executive functioning abilities. Although Darrin met the criteria for ADHD, use of psycho-stimulants such as Ritalin that might otherwise treat ADHD were not found effective. The reason was quite simple. Darrin lacked the necessary brain cells upon which the medications might have otherwise worked. Newer neuroimaging tests such as PET and SPECT scanning that can show actual cell activity may allow for better diagnoses in the future, but at this time, they are very expensive, and even less likely to be currently used in a person with disabilities.

3. Even though a person can be clinically diagnosed as having a certain disorder, the medications currently at hand have never been tested in persons with various structural abnormalities of the brain. The appropriate medications, dosages, and the expected responses are not understood in a research sense and could only be discovered in a clinical setting. Unfortunately this lack of specific knowledge can result in many medication difficulties for the individual and for those around them.

Those difficulties aside, however, we must continue to forge ahead in our abilities to assess, diagnose and treat some of these devastating psychiatric disorders.

The Diagnostic and Statistical Manual IV-TR (DSM IV-TR), (2000) is a cookbook collection of the best-defined psychiatric disorders. Key criteria issues along with several others commonly found symptoms typically define the diagnoses. The person will have to meet a certain number of the criteria in order for the diagnosis to be made. Because people with developmental disabilities frequently have difficulty with communication, or at least practitioners may not be able to understand their form of communication, psychiatric diagnoses have been deemed difficult at best to determine.

Consider, however, the DSM IV-TR criteria for major depression (Chart 4.2). You will realize that the criteria can easily be adapted and understood in persons with disabilities. For example, the individual may not say that he no longer enjoys favorite activities, but you will notice that he refuses to go bowling. She may not say that she cannot fall asleep, but you may see her wandering around the group home until 1 AM. Chart 4.3 is a mood scale based on DSM IV-TR criteria that helps to gather initial information and follow a person's mood.

Unlike a lot of other baseline type charts that you have probably filled out somewhere, "0" is not necessarily baseline for the person being monitored. The person's "baseline" may actually be a -2 on a highly regular basis.

Symptoms of Major Depression (DSM IV-TR)

Must include:
- Depressed (may appear as irritable) mood.

OR • Loss of interest or pleasure.

In addition, four or more of the following symptoms must be present during the same two-week period:
- Significant weight change (without trying).
- Insomnia or over-sleeping.
- Restlessness or significant loss of movement.
- Fatigue, loss of energy.
- Feelings of worthlessness or excessive guilt.
- Decreased ability to concentrate or indecisiveness.
- Recurrent thoughts of death or suicide.

Chart 4.2

"0" equals euthymic (happy, content) mood for anybody. At "0", people smile appropriately. They enjoy and engage in activities. They interact well with others. They sleep seven to nine hours per night without difficulty. Their appetite is stable, and their concentration is appropriate to their functioning level. That's just basic mood. It's where we all hope to fit most of the time. A lot of us tend to fluctuate between the "-1"and the "+1" and that's okay too. Don't go diagnosing yourself here! For people with depression, however, a –1 may actually be an "up" day for them.

Let's go back to our friends the little neurotransmitters in figure 4.1. In the case of major depression, the most commonly implicated neurotransmitter is still Serotonin. If, and *for example only*, it takes 100 serotonins to complete the signal transmission from Cell #1 to Cell #2, someone with major depression may only be providing 50 to 60 little serotonins to the second cell. This creates as efficient of a system as trying to run an eight-cylinder car on five cylinders. The car doesn't run well if at all. When the individual nerve cells in the brain do not produce enough of the serotonin or at the very least not enough is getting onto the next cell, the person will not feel well, regardless of that person's strength of character, moral fiber, or number of smacks upside the head. Punches to the stomach won't cure diabetes; smacks upside the head won't cure depression either.

Hopelessness that life can ever get any better is not only common, but also a key indicator in depression. Crying and despondent facial features are behavioral cues of hopelessness. If hopelessness is not expressed or easily determined, a person can still be diagnosed with depression if they have anhedonia, or lack of enjoyment in previously enjoyed activities.

Looking back at the mood scale, let's say that Donna is at a "-1" on the scale. When staff announces an outing by saying, "Come on! We're going shopping. We are going

The Mood Chart
(Chart 4.3a)

Name: _____

Month/Year: _____

Circle the appropriate number that corresponds with the individual's mood/behavior for the day. Please keep seperate logs for home and school/day activity.

+3	severe mania
+2	moderate mania
+1	mild mania
0	normal mood
-1	mild depression
-2	moderate depression
-3	severe depression

DATE		SCHOOL/DAY LOG								HOME/NIGHT LOG					
1	+3	+2	+1	0	-1	-2	-3	+3	+2	+1	0	-1	-2	-3
2	+3	+2	+1	0	-1	-2	-3	+3	+2	+1	0	-1	-2	-3
3	+3	+2	+1	0	-1	-2	-3	+3	+2	+1	0	-1	-2	-3
4	+3	+2	+1	0	-1	-2	-3	+3	+2	+1	0	-1	-2	-3
5	+3	+2	+1	0	-1	-2	-3	+3	+2	+1	0	-1	-2	-3
6	+3	+2	+1	0	-1	-2	-3	+3	+2	+1	0	-1	-2	-3
7	+3	+2	+1	0	-1	-2	-3	+3	+2	+1	0	-1	-2	-3
8	+3	+2	+1	0	-1	-2	-3	+3	+2	+1	0	-1	-2	-3
9	+3	+2	+1	0	-1	-2	-3	+3	+2	+1	0	-1	-2	-3
10	+3	+2	+1	0	-1	-2	-3	+3	+2	+1	0	-1	-2	-3
11	+3	+2	+1	0	-1	-2	-3	+3	+2	+1	0	-1	-2	-3
12	+3	+2	+1	0	-1	-2	-3	+3	+2	+1	0	-1	-2	-3
13	+3	+2	+1	0	-1	-2	-3	+3	+2	+1	0	-1	-2	-3
14	+3	+2	+1	0	-1	-2	-3	+3	+2	+1	0	-1	-2	-3
15	+3	+2	+1	0	-1	-2	-3	+3	+2	+1	0	-1	-2	-3
16	+3	+2	+1	0	-1	-2	-3	+3	+2	+1	0	-1	-2	-3
17	+3	+2	+1	0	-1	-2	-3	+3	+2	+1	0	-1	-2	-3
18	+3	+2	+1	0	-1	-2	-3	+3	+2	+1	0	-1	-2	-3
19	+3	+2	+1	0	-1	-2	-3	+3	+2	+1	0	-1	-2	-3
20	+3	+2	+1	0	-1	-2	-3	+3	+2	+1	0	-1	-2	-3
21	+3	+2	+1	0	-1	-2	-3	+3	+2	+1	0	-1	-2	-3
22	+3	+2	+1	0	-1	-2	-3	+3	+2	+1	0	-1	-2	-3
23	+3	+2	+1	0	-1	-2	-3	+3	+2	+1	0	-1	-2	-3
24	+3	+2	+1	0	-1	-2	-3	+3	+2	+1	0	-1	-2	-3
25	+3	+2	+1	0	-1	-2	-3	+3	+2	+1	0	-1	-2	-3
26	+3	+2	+1	0	-1	-2	-3	+3	+2	+1	0	-1	-2	-3
27	+3	+2	+1	0	-1	-2	-3	+3	+2	+1	0	-1	-2	-3
28	+3	+2	+1	0	-1	-2	-3	+3	+2	+1	0	-1	-2	-3
29	+3	+2	+1	0	-1	-2	-3	+3	+2	+1	0	-1	-2	-3
30	+3	+2	+1	0	-1	-2	-3	+3	+2	+1	0	-1	-2	-3
31	+3	+2	+1	0	-1	-2	-3	+3	+2	+1	0	-1	-2	-3

The Mood Chart Key

Circle the most appropriate number for the day. Pick the larger number when 2 or more items apply for the individual that day. **Note: A person is rarely "very depressed" and "very manic" on the same day. If a mood shifts this rapidly, the person is LABILE.

+3 Constant motion, frequently in danger to self or others, appears unable to stop, speech is very fast/pressured, requires less than 4 hours sleep, and does not appear tired. May require hospitalization at this point.

+2 Extremely active, difficult to maintain focus, acts out without provocation and almost seems to enjoy being in trouble. Eats very fast or not at all. Grandiose, often labile or very irritable mood.

+1 More active, more energy than usual, but not out of control. May need less sleep (1-2 hours less). Seems more "upbeat" than would be expected, easily distracted.

0 Smiles appropriately, enjoys and engages in activities, interacts well with others, sleeps 7-9 hours per night without difficulty, appetite is stable. Concentration appropriate to functioning level.

-1 Appears sad much of the time, does not appear to enjoy activities, but will participate with encouragement. Often tired or restless. Change in appetite.

-2 Cries frequently. Will not engage in activities or conversations. Avoids people, isolates. Sleep is altered. Decrease in self-care activities/tolerance. Poor concentration. Reduced motor movements. Easily agitated, hopeless, expresses guilt.

-3 Talks of death (self/others). Frequent/severe injury to self/others. Does not respond to any successful prompts to redirect behavior.

to the mall. Joe needs underwear. (Won't that be an exciting shopping trip!?) Come on Donna, we're leaving." She doesn't leap up at the prospect. Staff asks a number of times and with each successive time their tone increases and their manners decrease. Finally, just because Donna is tired of hearing staff, she will stand up and slowly meander her way on downstairs ready to get into the van. At the mall, she lags behind the rest of the group. She is attending the activity and this will look nice on the charts, but she is clearly not having a good time.

When I am conducting an evaluation of an individual with potential depression, I ask the individual to tell me the last thing that she enjoyed. Before I start this line of questioning, I often have to put a gag order on the staff persons attending the assessment. If allowed time to simply come up with something of her own that she last enjoyed, several minutes of agonizing silence will probably follow. Finally, because many of the people that I have evaluated have been taught to be far too compliant, they will come up with something like, "Um, I like bowling."

If I then inquire as to the last time she actually asked to go bowling, I may find out that she hasn't bowled in over a year. Now, I myself last bowled a whopping "36 points" (and this was bumper bowling), and understand not wanting to go bowling. But for this individual who might otherwise enjoy it, finding out that she has refused to bowl once staff insists she go to the bowling alley is a major piece of information. (We must separate out boredom with an activity from lack of enjoyment.) The reason I ask staff not to speak is that frequently staff will point out the various activities that the person was involved in. As in Donna's case, I didn't ask what she was involved in; I asked what she enjoyed. Remember attending your spouse's high school reunion? You complied and attended, but did you truly enjoy it?

Continuing on, a person at "-1" appears tired or restless much of the time. You might start to notice sleep disturbances that will increase as the depression worsens. There is either an increase or decreased interest in food. Most typically people who are mildly depressed will have an increased interest in food (perhaps in relationship to the anxiety felt). People who are more severely depressed will often have a decreased interest in food. It is not uncommon to see a change of weight over the past three month period in excess of 10 to 20 pounds.

Let's say that Donna is now at a "-2". She cries frequently (hopelessness?) for no apparent reason or seemingly irrelevant reasons. She will not engage in activities that used to be enjoyed or even enforced. Donna tends to put herself in a corner. If she lives in a place where she is not allowed into her bedroom during "program time", she will find a place to isolate herself. She will not participate in activities and if you try to get her to participate in activities, you can begin counting the aggressive episodes for the month. Because the aggression seems linked to requests for her to participate, we may erroneously consider the aggression as a severe form of "non-compliance."

Did you know that people with disabilities have aggression that "comes out of the blue?" I know this because I have sat in on any number of assessments where I have heard that very statement. As we began to better understand the relationship between aggression and upsetting events within the environment, people worked harder and harder to try to find out why the aggression occurred. Frequently, however, we simply don't have a total understanding of what has gone on (and their emotional reaction to those events) in that person's day or even in that person's week that would give rise to the understanding of the aggression we are currently seeing.

Perhaps you never have a bad day but I have been known to have them on occasion. I'm out of clean blue jeans and am reduced to nothing clean, but my lone business suit. I get a speeding ticket on my way to work. My desk is overrun with papers. I am late getting home from work and the kids are hungry, each with after-school activities that they need to be to in one hour. I then remember that I was supposed to get bread and milk on my way home, and I forgot to thaw out anything. Dreading the thought of fast-food (again), I frantically search the refrigerator for any leftover left-overs; there are none.

On the way to the drive-thru, the children remind me: A.) One classroom had been promised homemade cookies by tomorrow and B.) I had promised the other child to help her correct her 10-page report. Pulling out of the drive-thru, the children knock my arm and I spill ketchup on my dry-clean-only suit and realize I never even had a chance to get out of the panty hose. I scream.

In my best June Cleaver voice, I quietly explain to the children that they must refrain from unexpected movements in a 1-ton projectile missile going 60 miles an hour down the road. At least that's what I hope I said and sounded like. I suspect if you ask my children, it sounded entirely different. To my children, my verbal acts of aggression at this point seemed "out of the blue". To those of you who can relate to my day, my outburst does not seem unusual, perhaps not even unreasonable, and certainly not "out of the blue".

Unfortunately, the people with whom we work frequently deal with the ever-changing world of shift change and staff turnover. What one staff person may have understood about John's day, the next staff person may not. When John walks past Pat who 'accidentally' sticks out his foot and John falls, we wonder why John pummels Pat. We assume that John's aggression is "out of the blue". What we don't understand is that Pat has spent the last eight hours at program causing John to trip and fall and John had had enough.

John's aggression was no more "out of the blue" than my episode was. I tried explaining to my children that I won second place in the meanest mom contest last year (when you are in second place you try harder), but I truly don't justify yelling irrationally at my children, but sometimes the day happens. I then have to apologize. In John's case, compound this occasional day into weeks, months or even years of hopeless living. For the person with depression, the feeling of being overwhelmed and irritable occur daily, not just once and a while. Undiagnosed, the irritability seems unreasonable to the ones around them. Thus comes the frustration and desire to "smack them upside the head".

While noticeable in the milder stages of depression, a very common symptom in deeper depression is a sleep disturbance. Most common are problems falling asleep, staying asleep, or waking too early in the morning. It is not unusual to see all these in one person. Have you ever had trouble falling asleep one night? You might be very nervous about something going on the next day and you watch the clock go by 11:30, 12:00, 12:30, and 1:00. You know you have to get up at 6:00 a.m. regardless of what time you fall asleep. You feel like screaming at this point. Staff will often report to me that Fred is up until 2:00 a.m. tearing his room apart and making so much noise, no one else can sleep. It is the same thing as your occasional night without sleep; except for the depressed person it is a nightly occurrence.

You're thinking, "Yeah, but I don't tear the room up." See, caught you! This is true, but you can work out your frustrations by thinking about tearing the room up! Particularly when a person is nonverbal, they act out their frustration in behavioral acts. Actually, even though I can be too verbal, some days my vocabulary just doesn't serve me the way a slammed door, a banged table or throwing things about my room can.

People with a sleep disturbance have a problem that causes frustration and requires care. It is not a function of their level of abilities, nor do they plan to upset your day. Depression is not the only cause of a sleep disturbance. If someone you care about (never you personally, I'm sure) sounds like Smoky the Bear or a chain saw in full gear when they sleep, this may be a sign of a physical sleep disturbance. The most common of these is sleep apnea. People with sleep apnea have episodes of very loud snoring with periods of dead silence in between. These quiet times are actually periods when the person with sleep apnea is NOT breathing! As we discussed earlier, lack of oxygen to the brain is a serious problem. People who are overweight or persons with Down syndrome are quite prone to sleep apnea. Over time, the person with sleep apnea will appear exhausted, unmotivated, and irritable. Antidepressants will not help here, but other interventions will.

Nevertheless, if you suspect depression or some other sleep disturbance in someone you care about or for, record sleep data for at least 2 weeks if not a full month on a chart such as 4.4. Take this chart with you when the evaluation of concerns occurs. Important points to record include the time a person goes to bed, what time he actually falls asleep, number and length of nighttime awakenings, and time that the person wakes in the morning. If possible, it is also good to record the amount of time spent napping per day/week as well.

After the initial visit with Diane and her mother, Diane (who could independently tell time) was asked to keep a record of sleep. Diane started by putting down the time she went to bed, what time she fell asleep, and how many times she woke up during the night. The final mark was when she woke up. Like Diane, some people with depression try to sleep in excess of 8 to 10 hours per day. When looking closer, however, what we will frequently find out is that they are lying in bed but they are not

The Sleep Chart
(Chart 4.4)

Name: _____

Month/Year: _____

1. Place an "A" in the box if the individual is **Awake** for any time during the indicated 30 minute time period.
2. Place a "B" in the box when the person initially went to **Bed**.
3. Place a "U" in the box when he/she got **Up** the next day.

DATE	9:00 PM	9:30	10:00	10:30	11:00	11:30	midnight	12:30	1:00	1:30	2:00	2:30	3:00	3:30	4:00	4:30	5:00	5:30	6:00	6:30	7:00	7:30	8:00	8:30	9:00 AM
1																									
2																									
3																									
4																									
5																									
6																									
7																									
8																									
9																									
10																									
11																									
12																									
13																									
14																									
15																									
16																									
17																									
18																									
19																									
20																									
21																									
22																									
23																									
24																									
25																									
26																									
27																									
28																									
29																									
30																									
31																									

actually sleeping this entire time. Even after eight to ten hours of being in bed, they don't feel rested.

One of the biggest complaints from people with sleep disturbances is the nighttime awakenings that occur. Those of you who have had children will recall bandaged sleep. When our children were being nursed, my husband quickly figured out that I was the only one with the supplies and equipment that could adequately feed them during the night. Therefore, his need to wake up during the night was minimal. Since he was working full time and I was home with the children, this seemed a reasonable expectation... at least for the first night. What I discovered in my daytime cherubs, however, is that those little monsters wanted to eat every 1 ½ to 2 hours during the night. Even though I might net an entire eight hours sleep somewhere in the 24-hour period, when it was bandaged together in between episodes of nursing; it just never felt like I got enough sleep.

We now know through science that adults need at least 90 to 120 minutes of uninterrupted sleep in order to make it through a complete sleep cycle. Most adults need 3-4 complete sleep cycles, hence the 7 – 9 hours required. Inability to go through these sleep cycles (no surprise to moms) can truly turn us psychotic.

Programmed sleep disturbances are a too common issue, but some don't even recognize it exists! I remember in nursing school learning that if someone was immobile or incontinent, they should be repositioned/changed every

2 hours – night or day. Unfortunately, staff's 2-hour schedule does not necessarily correlate to the person's sleep cycle. Stage 3 sleep is the very deep, restorative sleep vital to human healing and growth. When we interrupt this stage, we were basically creating sleep disturbances in people that might otherwise not have had them. Group homes will want to consider alternative options when they have residents who are incontinent. Use of ultra absorbant diapering materials and other plastic protective devises will allow people to enjoy blissful sleep for at least 3 ½ to 4 hours at a time. People will be happier simply because they are getting quality sleep.

When a person is suffering from depression, they are also lacking adequate stage 3 sleep as a function of the depression. Many older prescription sleep agents, and even diphenhydramine (found in Benadryl and many over the counter sleep agents) help a person fall asleep, ands stay asleep, but they may still miss out on adequate amounts of stage 3 sleep as well as experience morning "hangover". The lack of effective sleep compounds with the other symptomatology of depression to make the entire picture worse. It is this disturbance of sleep that often prompts most people to first seek help.

Diane had a decrease in self-care activities. In a word, I was glad I met her in winter, because in summer, the body odor would have been overwhelming. Sometimes, the person with depression is limited in the ability to bathe and groom. The person, who requires help with bathing/grooming, often won't allow other people to do it for him either. The staff person may be appropriately trying to help him brush his teeth, but the depressed person is smacking staff out of the way. This appears on the aggression charts as acts 13, 17, & 20 of the month while in reality several issues could be at play here.

Number one, like Diane, people who are depressed typically don't take care of themselves that well. On the day when I am not feeling particularly red hot, I don't get all dressed up. I don't bother with makeup and I lounge around in my old grubby blue jeans, sweatshirt, and old tennis shoes. Days when I am feeling good, I get dressed up. I may actually put on some "chapstick" and my good blue jeans, sweater, and good tennis shoes. When you are depressed, there is the feeling that you don't even deserve to look nice on ANY day because you are not worthy of it. You may even go so far as to rip up the new clothes that someone just bought you.

A second issue needs to be taken into account. When somebody is aggressive particularly in the area of self-care, we need to remember that this person may have been abused. During times of self-care may have been when the abuser had free access to assault the victim. Don't forget to ask all the questions that need to be asked. The abuse doesn't have to be happening now for the reactions to be occurring now.

Even if not abused, having to allow others intimate contact is difficult at best. When my parents first married, my mother tripped down a flight of stairs. She had both arms in casts. She said that the most difficult part was allowing even loved family members to perform intimate self-care acts such as wiping after toileting. After years of nursing, I am still amazed at the people who have allowed me, a stranger, to assist them with necessary activities. When I taught nursing students in a nursing home, I was never surprised when on occasion a person who had lost verbal skills acted "aggressive". They were saying "No." in the only way left to them.

It is a sad reality that many group homes have a rapid turnover of staff. When a person with multiple disabilities requires physical assistance with self care in a group home, that person may have staff that they have never met before coming in and helping with private matters. If the person has been abused before, they won't know by the nametag if that staff person can be trusted or not. The person acting violent in this scenario may or may not be depressed. One symptom does not equal a diagnosis.

Still on the same old mood chart, continuing at a –2, the person may experience an increase (fidgety, restless pacing, etc.) or decrease (very slow movement or no movement) in motor activity. In addition, the depressed person's ability to stay on task (concentrate) is much less than usual. When my father passed away, no one was surprised that my work suffered for a time from grief. I recovered, but depressed persons are rarely able to work up to their potential. In 1990, in the United States alone, the annual cost of depression was 44 billion dollars...much of this in lost productivity. The Canadian <u>Globe and Mail</u>

had a special edition on mental illness on June 12, 2000. By this point, figures were estimated at 80 billion (US) dollars in lost productivity, of which 2/3 was a result of depression.

At a "-3" on the mood chart, the person talks of death either of themselves or others a lot. Now obviously this criterion is for people who are verbal. I also want to distinguish this from those individuals who have had a relatively recent loss because then talk of death is appropriate. During my dad's funeral, people talked of other losses they have known whether it was animals, family members, friends or jobs. When a loss is experienced, people will bring up other losses that they are still dealing with. This is normal grieving. And please note, just because we think it was a wonderful opportunity for a group home staff to get promoted to a supervisory position in another group home, it still meant another loss in a long chain of losses for the individual left at the old group home. People who are severely depressed, however, will talk of death frequently...with or without recent losses.

For people with major depression, life often seems so hopeless and bleak that the desire to be dead is quite prevalent. Suicide has not, however, been as serious a concern in persons with disabilities. The reasons for this may have to do more with the limited cognitive abilities and the structured living situations that many persons with intellectual challenges find themselves in as opposed to the presence or absence of a desire to be dead. Lack of access to lethal methods and presence of others are known deterrents to suicide for all people.

Death is an abstract thought. Persons with mental retardation may not have the concept of death as an escape or as a way out but they certainly feel the pain and the hurt and the self-inflicted aggression may be a function of this.

As you can tell, people with major depression are in the pits. They can be severely aggressive. They can be seriously self injurious. Even when they are not aggressive or self-injurious, they are significantly unhappy. They will not participate. This is not non-compliance. This is a treatable illness called depression. There is no behavior treatment plan that is going to get those little transmitters moving again not even if you dole tokens out along the way with little smacks upside the head.

So if smacks upside the head don't work, what will? The treatment options most frequently used for major depression include medications and psychotherapy. Some of the first medications used for depression are still used today. The heterocyclic (and tricyclics) antidepressants that are still in use include Elavil and Pamelor (see chart 4.5a). Although frequently effective medications, many practitioners choose not to prescribe them because of their side effect profile.

Common side effects of the tricyclic medications include excessive drowsiness and constipation. For older people, there is also a big problem with standing too quickly and becoming dizzy. This is called orthostatic hypotension.

---

*Older Antidepressant Medications**

amitriptyline	Elavil	75 - 200 mg/day
amoxapine	Asendin	75 - 200 mg/day
desipramine	Norpramin	75 - 200 mg/day
imipramine	Tofranil	75 - 200 mg/day
nortriptyline	Pamelor	25 - 150 mg/day

Common side effects include - Low blood pressure, dry mouth, urinary retention, blurry vision, confusion, constipation, sexual dysfunction and weight gain.

Monoamine Oxidase Inhibitors (MAOI's) - Rarely used.

phenelzine	Nardil	15 - 75 mg/day
tranylcypromine	Parnate	10 - 40 mg/day

Note - There must be a 2 - 6 week delay between taking other antidepressants and an MAOI. MAOI's can cause a severe hypertensive crisis.

* Only a partial listing.

Chart 4.5a

Your blood stays in the feet but your head is dangling up in the air without enough oxygen running around to help you function. Clearly when somebody already has a gait disturbance or difficulty moving around, sudden dizziness while standing up provides too much of a chance of a fractured hip.

The good news isn't over yet. Other side effects can include skin reactions such as allergic rash or easy sun burning. Sunscreen is a must for these people. There are also potential changes in the white blood cells (infection fighters) and platelets (for blood clotting). Not only that, sexual difficulties, anxiety, insomnia, increased appetite and weight, and increased risk for seizure activity can also occur. Along with these side effects is the potential risk for overdosing on these medications for people still feeling suicidal! For several decades, these medications were the best options for folks with depression, causing some people to wonder, which was worse, the illness or the treatment.

Another class of medications still in use is the <u>MAO inhibitors</u> (unless you are on "Jeopardy", you will probably never need to know what those letters stand for). Although effective in the treatment of major depression, many practitioners avoid them because of the mandatory dietary restrictions. Persons taking MAO inhibitors must avoid foods high in the amino acid (the building blocks of proteins) tyramine. Foods high in tyramine include red wine, aged cheeses, yogurt and vinegar. The whole list is rather lengthy and restrictive in terms of food choices. MAO inhibitors cannot be taken with many other medications including over-the-counter medicines. If these foods or medicines are eaten while on an MAO inhibitor, the person can experience a tyramine crisis, which causes extremely elevated blood pressure, possibly a stroke or even death. There must also be a two-week to two-month drug free period between these medications and any other antidepressants. Therefore if these medications don't work, there will be at least two weeks before another medication can be tried and several more weeks before these medicines start to be effective.

Currently, the preferred drugs of choice for depression are the (chart 4.5b) <u>selective serotonin re-uptake inhibitors (SSRI's)</u>. How's that for a mouthful? Knowing what SSRI's stand for is wonderful if you ever must answer the $800 dollar question on "Jeopardy", but otherwise simply understanding the broad category is enough for most people. If we look back on our little nerve cells (chart 4.1), we realize that nerve cells are very environmentally conscious and recycle. When a signal needs to be transmitted from one nerve cell to the other, cell number one spits out the correct neurotransmitter. In this case we are talking about Serotonin. After the neurotransmitters have been released out into the space between the cells, and used by the second cell, they get sucked back up by the nerve cells for reuse. What the SSRI's are reported to do **over time** is prevent the re-uptake of the Serotonin, so that there is more Serotonin available in this space. Over a period of time, even if cell number one still only releases 50% of the necessary transmitter, there is extra Serotonin available to complete the signal (hence the name, reuptake inhibitor). As time went on, scientists recognized that the SSRI's caused other chemical changes in the brain. They also act to reregulate other cell activities vital to the overall function of the brain including promoting correct release and transfer of other chemicals as well as regulate the number of connection ports (receptors).

Hopefully by now the observant reader has noted that I said these medications have their effect "over a period of time". Although some of the newer antidepressants are claiming to start working as fast as one week, it still re-

Chart 4.5b

generic name	brand name	dose range (mg / day)	sedation	inital activation	GI upset	sexual dysfunction	sweating
citalopram	Celexa	20 - 40	X		X	X X	
escitalopram	Lexapro	10 - 20			X	X	
fluoxetine	Prozac	5 - 60		X X	X	X X	X
fluvoxamine	Luvox	50 - 300			X X	X X	
paroxetine	Paxil	10 - 50	X X		X X	X X	X
paroxetine	Paxil CR	12.5 - 37.5	X		X	X X	X
sertraline	Zoloft	25 - 200		X	X	X X	X
trazodone	Desyrel	50 - 300	X X			X priapism	

SSRI: Selective Serotonin Receptor Inhibitor

All have the potential to lower seizure threshold, induce mania in persons with Bipolar D/O, headaches, serotonin syndrome.

quires most agents at least 2-6 weeks for any significant improvement to be noted. While it can take up to a month before helpful effects are noted, side effects can occur immediately. This makes the prescribing and use of these medications very difficult.

I went into nursing and psychiatric nursing in specific with the general idea of helping people feel better. As my husband will quickly point out, patience has never been my long suit. When I see somebody in pain, I want to help her feel better quickly. Unfortunately, changing brain chemistry doesn't happen as fast as our fast food society would like it to. When I take aspirin for my headache, I don't want to wait a month for it to work; I want my headache gone within 30 to 60 minutes. As annoying as chronic sinus headaches can be, the pain involved pales compared to the pain associated with major depression. The wait is often hard causing many people to quit or find their own more immediate relief such as illicit drug and alcohol usage (which serve to significantly worsen symptoms after a very short time) or even suicide.

When the SSRI's first came out, they were hailed as the medications with very few side effects. Unfortunately, reality over time has informed us that this is not entirely true. The side effect profiles, however, are still much more favorable compared to the older antidepressants, but no medication is without its faults.

Prozac is considered by many to be the Kleenex of the industry. Kleenex is a brand name for paper tissues that we all use during cold season. Many refer to all paper tissues as Kleenex because that was the brand that we all know. This is true with many things such as gelatin being referred to as Jell-O, etc. Just like my husband and the coffee mug, Prozac is what everyone stops to think about when one thinks of an antidepressant.

The most common initial side effect to fluoxetine (Prozac) is stimulation. This is much like one would feel after a strong cup of coffee – with or without the mug. Since many people with depression lack energy, this can be a good thing. It is advisable, however, to take it in the morning. Amazingly, improved sleep is generally the first sign that these medications are working. There is the occasional person whom Prozac will make drowsy, and in this case these people should take it in the evening before bedtime. The tendency towards activation can also be seen with Zoloft (sertraline), and perhaps Luvox (fluvoxamine) and Celexa (citalopram). On the other hand, Desyrel (Trazodone) and Paxil (paroxetine) have a tendency towards sedation and are best taken at night. Paxil is also associated with some mild stomach upset for the first one to two weeks and is best taken with milk or food. Paxil CR (controlled release) may minimize these side effects. In general, however, for all of them, the side effects are generally milder and better tolerated than those with the older medications.

The SSRI's can also have an effect on sexuality. Since many depressed people are not interested in sexual activity, this side effect may not be reported or noted at first.

As the depression lifts, however, their libido should return. Unfortunately the medications can commonly cause delayed ejaculation and sometimes inability to achieve orgasm in both men and women. Some people even say that while they are no longer depressed, they are dismayed with their lack of interest or response to sex. Imagine feeling better, but either feeling no sexual excitement towards your partner or being unable to experience either (or both) orgasm or ejaculation. "Hey doc, can't I just be just a little bit depressed so I can be excited!?" Since there are ways to deal with this problem, please remember to let your practitioner know if you or someone you care about is having these sorts of problems. Indeed, all side effects, no matter, how mild should be reported so that the practitioner can better help you.

More than one transmitter is implicated in depression. The SSRI's alone may not provide adequate relief for all people. The medicines that act on norepinephrine, another neurochemical associated with depression, alone or in combination with the SSRI's may be more effective. Two such antidepressants (chart 4.5c) that are dispensed as a combo are Effexor and Effexor XR (venlafaxine), and nefazodone (brand name Serzone, pulled from the market spring 2004). Paxil in higher dosages also impacts on both the serotonin and norepinephrin systems. Effexor is associated with a significant amount of nausea and vomiting and again is recommended to be taken with food. Since it has recently come out in an extended release (XR) format, it may only need to be taken once a day with less stomach upset as opposed to two to three times a day as when it was first released. Nefazodone has been associated with more sedation than other newer antidepressants and must be taken twice a day, which makes it difficult for some people. Serzone (previous brand name for nefazodone) was also recently "black-boxed" by the US FDA for potentially dangerous liver complications. It is now to be used only under careful observation. One of the positive attributes of nefazodone, however, is its action on serotonin is different such that it is not associated with sexual side effects.

There are two other current antidepressants with unique characteristics. Wellbutrin (buproprion) actually works on different neurotransmitters such as dopamine. It is a very effective antidepressant however. It is also used in the treatment of ADHD (especially if depression and ADHD exist together). While its effects on ADHD are not immediate like Ritalin, it can be very effective. It too does not seem to impact sexuality, and may even help with sexual side effects associated with the SSRI's. Occasional mild appetite suppression and even weight loss may be seen with Wellbutrin. Buproprion was also released under the trade name of Zyban, which is used for smoking cessation.

When Wellbutrin was first released, prior to the "SR" and "XL" versions, initial drug trials indicated a serious risk of seizures. Since all antidepressants run the risk of lowering the seizure threshold, (That is, the person is more likely to have seizures if they have a seizure disorder.) one must be cautious about any antidepressants when

Other Antidepressants
Chart 4.5c

Clomipramine (Anafranil) 25 - 250 mg/day.
  Primarily used for OCD.
  Side effects include: sedation, constipation, tremor, dizziness, sexual
  dysfunction, sweating, dry mouth, weight gain, blurred vision

buproprion (Wellbutrin, Wellbutrin SR, ZYBAN) 200 - 450 mg/day
  Also used for ADHD, and "Zyban" for smoking cessation.
  Causes little or no sedation, heart problem, or sexual dysfunction.
  Side effects include: Greater potential risk of seizure, agitation,
  initial anxiety, insomnia, decreased appetite, dry mouth.

mirtazapine (Remeron) 7.5 - 45 mg/day
  side effects: extreme sedation, especially at low dosage, weight
  gain, need to check liver enzymes, dry mouth

nefazodone 200 - 600 mg/day
  side effects: sedation, dry mouth, constipation, dizziness, GI upset,
  little or no sexual dysfunction. [Black box warning by FDA.]

Venlafaxine (Effexor XR) 75 - 225 mg/day
            (Effexor) 75 - 350 g/day
  Side effects: GI upset, dizziness, sedation, dry mouth, sweating,
  sexual dysfunction, weight gain

the person also has seizures. I know of many people with both seizures and depression and both are adequately treated, but care must be exercised in treatment. Current studies of Wellbutrin SR and XL do not seem to show any greater risk of seizures than other antidepressants, but many practitioners remain cautious.

Remeron (mirtazapine) is believed to work unlike the tricyclics, or SSRI's. It seems to have its effects on the norepinephrine channels of the brain, (which in turn effect serotonin). Because it actually calms the stomach, it has been used with chemotherapy. In some people, it also seems to increase a person's appetite, which helps with possible weight gain. Although I certainly don't need it, there are those people with severe depression for whom this initial side effect is helpful. Another unique characteristic is sedation associated with dosage. Most medications that cause sedation have increasing sedation when you increase the dosage. With Remeron, people will feel the most sedation at 7.5 – 15 mg./day, and little sedation at the usual dose of 30 mg.!

St. John's Wort is a substance sold in health food stores, grocery stores, and even "dollar" stores here in the United States. It is described by some as "Nature's Prozac." Unlike Prozac, an SSRI, St. John's Wort is actually an MAO Inhibitor and should never be taken with other antidepressants. Although the active ingredient, 3% Hypercin has been used extensively in Europe and Canada for depression, the US FDA has not approved it for use here in the US.

At this time there are several serious concerns with its usage. Because the FDA has not released study data on this drug, standard dosages, interactions, and side effects are not listed anywhere on the label. While I'm sure this information is out there in cyberspace, how many of us look up that data on our daily multivitamin? People treat SJW like a vitamin, but like the other antidepressants; It can have serious interactions with other medications yet people may not remember to report taking it to their practitioners.

As SJW is not treated as a medication, fillers are also not regulated. All medications have active ingredients, and then are held together with "fillers". Generic equivalents of medicines must have similar fillers. Most people can tolerate generic acetaminophen for headaches as well as they do Tylenol (brand name of the same medicine). Since most older medicines (now including Prozac, Luvox and Paxil) have generic equivalents, they are often cheaper than newer or brand name medicines that are very important for people on a limited budget. I buy generic whenever possible. Not everyone can do this however.

Eric was a big guy. He was prescribed desipramine (an older tricyclic) for years. One month, the pharmacist gave him a different generic brand of the same medicine, but it was a different color. His mom noted almost immediately that he became agitated, irritable, and restless on the blue pill. She took it back to the pharmacist and demanded the white version back. His symptoms resolved in a few days. In this case, Eric was reacting to the usually indistinguishable differences between generic equivalents. This story sticks out because of the next saga.

I had been seeing Eric for over three years. His primary psychiatrist had seen him for several more years before that. This recent spring day, his mom reports that when the doctor started him on desipramine (4 years ago), she had seen a TV talk show on SJW. She had the desipramine prescription filled and bought a bottle of SJW and started them together. She felt the SJW was a natural supplement, and never thought to tell us when we asked each time if he was on any new medicines. For many people, mixing these 2 drug classes could have prompted a tyramine crisis seen with the prescribed MAO inhibitors. While in Eric's case the two have worked well together, what if she never told us and his desipramine was increased? Since the experience of the blue vs. white pills, Eric's mom has stayed with the same brand of SJW, but not everyone might stay with the same brand. Without regulations, greater discrepancies could occur than just blue vs. white. At this point, I cannot legally recommend St. Johns Wort here in the US; it is a case of buyer-beware!

When practitioners pick and chose a medication, we realize that at proper dosages, most of these medications are equally effective. That is, most people will experience relief from depression. The choosing of a particular medication has more to do with matching the potential additional benefits that each antidepressant may offer, such as improving sleep or treating co-existing anxiety, then direct superiority of any one medication over another.

We also try to match the potential side effect profile with what the person is likely to tolerate best. ALWAYS inform your practitioner of troublesome side effects you have ever had with other medications. For example, when one type of antibiotic caused severe stomach pain, my doctor avoids that whole class of antibiotics when I need one.

Care must be taken when adding medications together whether for psychiatric reasons or mixed with general physical medications. Through the complex system known as the cytochrome P450 system of the liver, better understood as the garbage disposal for the body, we are able to rid ourselves of foreign substances such as alcohol and medications. When any one port of the garbage disposal gets clogged up with too many things trying to go through it at once, a backlog of substances in the bloodstream occurs. This backlog can create medication toxicity or potentially harmful interactions between medications.

One piece of advice, as in the case of Eric, let all prescribing practitioners know of every other medication you or your person you are concerned about are taking including over the counter medications, vitamins, and even herbs sold at health food stores. I also strongly recommended you use one specific pharmacy so that that particular pharmacy's computer can recognize all the medications you are taking. Given the thousands of medications, both prescribed and over the counter, it is frequently the computer that will recognize potential interaction between medications and not the pharmacist or the practitioner.

People are often concerned because the have heard that various antidepressants cause suicide. Suicide is a concern, but for an unusual reason. One of the first signs that these medications are working is an improved sleep pattern. When a person begins to sleep better, they naturally have more energy. Some people become so immobilized from their depression that they literally don't have the energy to attempt suicide. One to two weeks after starting these medications can be the most critical time for suicide watch. In the olden days, people with severe depression particularly when suicidal were often hospitalized. Because people are now more commonly treated in the community, they are no longer professionally watched 24 hours a day during this critical one to two week period. The suicidal person in the community (or even in the hospital) now has more energy but they're not yet thinking clearly. This scenario can be true for all the antidepressants. Fortunately, not all people feel suicidal or with close monitoring come through this period unharmed.

There are other treatments for depression besides medications. Some centers continue to advocate for the use of electroconvulsive therapy or ECT. For people who are so resistant to current medications or so suicidal that time is critical, ECT may be a viable option. ECT has come a long way since the early days. At this time, persons are anesthetized and given electric charges to the brain. Literally, it is as if someone is jump-starting a dead battery on a cold morning. It is believed that the seizure-like activity activates the neurotransmitters and the mood elevation begins. Typical ECT treatments include 2 to 3 ECT's for 2 to 3 weeks. Some people require routine ECT treatments once every 2 to 4 weeks after that. The largest dangers to ECT include all of the risks associated with anesthesia, and some people experience amnesia about the ECT procedure, and occasionally amnesia regarding other events as well. It is also expensive since it must be done in a hospital setting, with physicians, anesthesiologists, etc.

Also effective for mild to moderate depression, in combination with the medications, are individual and group therapy. Therapy can be almost essential for people who have experienced long term depression. I remember listening to a psychiatrist comparing recovering from depression to somebody recovering from a stroke. When someone has had a stroke, it is not uncommon for him to lose function in one side of his body. We have come to realize that over time many stroke victims regain a fair amount of use back to their affected limbs. If, however, that limb did not receive therapy during the initial crisis, it would stiffen up and even though function might have returned from the inside out, because it is stiff the person no longer has use of it.

Let's take a look at somebody who has been severely depressed for a period of time. Their outlook on life is very hopeless and gloomy. They see themselves as failures, they see the world around them as never providing any hope, and the cup is eternally half empty. Even after the antidepressants have had an opportunity to work and the individual is sleeping better, they may enjoy some activities, and they may be more involved in their life, but their thought patterns are still stuck in a negative format.

Without the psychotherapy, to take a critical look at their thought patterns (formally referred to as cognitive behavioral therapy) people's thought patterns can be as stuck as the stroke victim's arm without physical therapy. When a person remains in negative thought patterns that go unchallenged, the lives of the family and friends surrounding the depressed person are often negatively impacted.

Regardless of the length of depression, therapy can be helpful to assist the person deal with painful realities in their past or present life. Sometimes, therapy alone is all that is necessary. Research has even documented brain chemical changes with therapy. Unfortunately, therapy is often a longer (read more expensive) form of help, and third party payers are hesitant to pay for it. If a person does not cope well with realities of life, however, medications alone will never completely assist the individual.

I realize that there are many people who believe that persons with developmental disabilities are incapable of insight and therefore could not benefit from therapy. But I assume that if you have read this far, you know better. As with all candidates for therapy, the starting point is assessment. You need to assess what the candidate feels the problems are, what you as the therapist foresee the problems to be, and (let's be real here) what the agency paying for the therapy perceives the problems to be. These three points rarely start off the same. Somewhere in the therapeutic process, the goals may begin to blend.

When I was assigned to Jessie in graduate school, her file was handed to me with a caution of "She has one MEAN attitude!" Jessie worried about independent living, she felt her primary concerns were threefold: (1) I'm bad; (2) Nobody likes me. And (3) I want a home of my own. From my standpoint, Jessie appeared depressed, had very little self-esteem, and had severely limited problem-solving skills. From an agency standpoint, she destroyed property, and was a physical threat to others in her home.

To describe a therapeutic process for individual or group therapy could be a book of its own. There are more therapeutic models to choose from than the grocery store has cereals. The secret to good relationships between consumers and therapists that I have seen seems to be the respect, acceptance, and honesty that both parties bring to the relationship. The ability to speak the same language is a nice luxury to start with, but not mandatory. As people grow in a relationship, they strive to understand each other's communication patterns.

People said to be "non-verbal" can also gain from a therapeutic process. Non-verbal does not mean non-communicating. Experts believe that 70% of most people's communication is non-verbal. Seventy percent is a lot to work with!!! Also, just because a person's mouth does not say words does not mean she doesn't hear. In fact, it may be quite useful to paraphrase with an individual what you suspect they may be feeling such as "I think I would feel angry if I see Fred getting a lot of Christmas presents and Christmas cards but my family never seems to send me anything." Statements such as this can go a long way towards helping the person understand that their internal feeling state is one of anger and that they have a right to feel anger. I would also couple this with the understanding that while it is understandable to feel angry, it is not okay to hit somebody else because I am angry.

Group therapy can be a helpful and cost effective form of therapy. In some cases, it can actually achieve more than individual therapy alone. One or two leaders can work with four to ten members in the same amount of time that each therapist could only see one person. Members gain support from each other. I have found that many persons with disabilities have been able to gain independent employment, move out on their own, and enjoy having the privacy. Unfortunately, over time, they also become quite lonesome without the network of peers from their group home or day program. Particularly for this group, the opportunity to socialize and develop friendships is an invaluable aspect of the group. People in a group begin to realize that others have experienced what they have. Members are often at different points of healing, such that they learn from each other.

At this time in my life, the clinic I work with serves almost 300 adults with dual diagnosis. Antidepressants are commonly prescribed. What seemed a routine evaluation for depression ended up being anything but. Ricky has severe mental retardation, and is essentially non-verbal. For the past 2-3 months, he had been lethargic, refusing to participate in usually enjoyed activities, and he was "sitting"! Staff assured me that Ricky, while not hyperactive, never just sat; he was always busy with something. He had been taken to an "urgent-care" clinic a few weeks ago, and diagnosed with the flu. The doctor there recommended an evaluation for depression. Since labs are routine, I ordered those before starting the anti-depressant I already had guardian consent for.

Ricky was hospitalized that afternoon with the lowest blood count I had ever seen outside of the hospital. He had a bleeding ulcer, and aspiration pneumonia. The consent was filed and never used.

Chapter 5

Bipolar Disorder:
A Roller Coaster Without An Amusement Park

Ecclesiastes 3:4a
"A Time To Weep And A Time To Laugh."

I hate roller coasters. A few summers ago, I had the dubious pleasure of going to a nationally known amusement park for the first time compliments of friends. Although only a four-hour drive from our home, I had never gone before. Considered "frugal" (or cheap, depending on who you are talking to), I have a basic disagreement with paying money so I can spin around on something metal and throw up. Since it was a free trip, the family overrode basic disagreement number one. Knowing I didn't like to spin and puke, the other family members informed me that I would certainly love the roller coasters. Even free, they were wrong.

The Park people pride themselves that these particular roller coasters have the ability to take you up to great heights and then smash you down to the lowest of ground in a mere matter of seconds. Some rides spin you upside down in circles while still going up and down. Some spin around blinding corners hundreds of feet above ground before the plummet. Another ride sinks into a blackened tunnel while jerking back and forth. All seemed hellish to me. After only 2 of these experiences which had the other 3 looking for more exciting rides, my greenish face and churning stomach spent the rest of the day in kiddy land. Thankfully, no more free tickets have come our way, so I haven't had to deal with these ups and downs. People with Bipolar Disorder, or manic-depression; however, live on a similar variety of emotional roller coasters – without tickets to get on or off.

Living on an incredibly fast emotional ride, Allen was a 47 year-old man diagnosed with severe mental retardation. He was at extreme risk of a one-way ticket back to the institution when I was called on consult. When I am sent out into the far corners of my state to evaluate "a problem", I can almost guarantee that the reason will be some variation of bipolar disorder. This particular day, after spending hours on snowy, ice-covered roads, was no exception. Though I was grateful to get to my destination alive, I can't say Allen was particularly thrilled to meet me. He spit at me, then ran out the door with 2 staff chasing behind him. This was certainly not the exercise portion of his behavior plan. Indeed, Allen was expected to participate in a work activity program, and then return home quietly to his adult foster care home.

Staff reported that for several days out of the week, Allen was non-stop high energy. He would get into a swing and pump wildly back and forth, back and forth, back and forth. He was in constant movement around the team space to the point where they had to put alarm systems on the door to make sure Allen didn't take off and head down the same icy roads that I had just traveled. On the same days that he was so busy at program, he would go home and sleep very little.

Fortunately for the AFC provider's sanity, after a few days of this non-stop activity, Allen would crash. Allen would crash to the extent that the homeowner had trouble getting him out of the house to go to program (thus giving program staff a break). During those days, he tried to sleep non-stop. He had been placed on a variety of medications with minimal success. Since Allen couldn't talk and didn't do the things others with "normal" IQ's might do, his symptoms had never been put together. Allen has a form of mixed state or even very rapid cycling Bipolar Disorder.

Closer to my home stomping grounds is a gentleman named Ron. Ron is the kind of guy I want with me when I have to travel to the less safe parts of town. He is big, strong, and he knows how to fight. Unfortunately, I know these things because staffs from his home and day program have placed many SOS calls to our office. For the first year that I knew him, I always saw him on the move. He seemed to enjoy getting into trouble (causing staff to often have raised blood pressures, as they KNEW it was behavioral!). He often started fights with his roommate. His roommate had untreated depression (later treated, once we realized Ron wasn't the whole problem) and tried to isolate himself. Ron would deliberately provoke him. Staff said, "He acts like he's staff!" Somedays he would refuse to eat, as he could not stop pacing. Ron is also essentially non-verbal with the exception of continuous singsong utterances. He was rumored to have profound retardation, but no one was sure. He wouldn't sit still long enough to be truly tested. He had been tried on countless behavioral plans along with Ritalin (for ADHD), Mellaril, and Haldol. Nothing seemed to help.

At the first appointment with his new psychiatrist, staffs were beside themselves. Ron had been going literally non-stop for over a week. He had been sleeping for less than two hours throughout these nights. Consequently none of the other people in his home had been sleeping for more than two to three hours as well. Paid and unpaid people alike, they were all becoming just a little bit irritable... and agitated as well.

A staff person from the home commented under his breath that he knew "at least Ron would soon stop. He was due for his 'shut down'." When asked to speak up, the staff person explained that after an extended period of agitation, Ron always collapsed for an equal length of time where he wouldn't move. Staffs were so grateful for the down times that they had never told the previous psychiatrist about them. Ron was also successfully treated for bipolar disorder.

Bipolar disorder I is the occurrence of one or more manic episodes or mixed episodes often with major depressive episodes (DSM IV-TR criteria for mania listed in Chart 5.1). Bipolar disorder II is the presence of one or more major depressive episodes with at least one episode of hypomania, but not a true manic or mixed episode. (A mixed episode is manic and depressive symptoms together.) These disorders generally hit people by their late teens/early twenties, but can begin later in life as well. The cycles can happen as rapidly as Allen's, that is, every three or four days from mania to depression. Or the cycles could extend as long as 20 years between the cycles of depression and mania. This wide variation in time spread often leads to confusion of accurate diagnosis. Suppose staff bring in a consumer who is acting "very wild", i.e. manic. If we don't have staff present to remember when he was depressed during the summer of 1989, the psychiatrist might miss the diagnosis of manic depression. In general, the earlier the onset, the more rapid the cycles, and the shorter time between cycles indicate greater severity of the illness, and the harder it is to achieve complete symptom relief.

> # Symptoms of a Manic Episode (DSM IV-TR)
>
> A. Distinct period of abnormally elevated, expansive, or irritable mood lasting at least one week or if hospitalized.
>
> B. Additionally, three or more of the following symptoms must be significantly exhibited:
>   - Inflated self-esteem or grandiosity.
>   - Decreased need for sleep.
>   - More talkaltive than usual, or pressured to keep talking (may be vocalizations, not necessarily words).
>   - Racing thoughts.
>   - Distractibility.
>   - Increased movements, agitation.
>   - Excessive pleasurable/dangerous activities.

Chart 5.1

To better understand mania, please look at the other half of the Mood Scale Chart 4.3 (pp. 65-66). At a +1, a person is more active than usual. He may have more energy, but is not out of control. Frankly these are often an enjoyable bunch of folks to invite to a party. They may need one to two hours less sleep. (Thus, they may offer to help clean up after the party!) Unlike people with depression who do not get enough sleep and are tired a lot, people with mania typically are not tired even with less sleep. The person with mania is usually upbeat, but some are more agitated than you would expect. They are easily distracted. They have difficulty completing tasks because they respond to any internal (i.e. hunger) or external (i.e. some one talking on the other side of the room) cue that prevails.

Level +1 on the mood scale is often difficult to differentiate from attention deficit disorder. Since it is not unusual to find ADHD during childhood in adults who go on to have bipolar disorder (and may continue to co-exist), and at this stage there are similarities, some people believe that attention deficit disorder (ADHD) and bipolar disorder may be on some type of continuum. This is for the researchers to debate.

People who are hypomanic (+1 - +2) on a continuous basis in the general population may not seek treatment on their own. Because they are lively and enjoy the constant rush of activities, they frequently don't see any problems in their lifestyle. Only when someone around them is severely disturbed by the constant activity and distraction, or the person is unable to complete work/school obligations will these people generally receive treatment of some sort. In addition, they may be involved in activities that could be viewed as somewhat dangerous or risky and this may also bring them to the attention of helpful authorities.

At a +2, people with mania are extremely active. They are difficult to keep on task in spite of constant supervision. They may act out without provocation and seem to enjoy being in trouble. This was the case of Ron who looked to his roommate for fights. These are the people who aggravate the daylights out of staff because they are forever getting into trouble. Unlike the depressed person off in the corner who only really gets aggressive if someone goes over and irritates him or her, the person with mania is out in the middle of the room causing trouble. As a matter of fact, like Ron, they are highly like to go over to the person in the corner and aggravate them because they know they can start a fight.

People with mania live on the edge—such that fighting and other high stimulation activities are preferred. It is not unusual to find out that the person is changing clothes every hour. She may begin wearing excessive make up. He may become sexually overactive often without the usual precautions. A common complaint is the massive unusual spending sprees. She may also consume large quantities of alcohol or illicit drugs or engage in other unsafe behaviors such as driving 90 miles an hour down an icy dirt road. In short, it is like having a wild college weekend all the time. This may even be the cause of unintentional suicide.

One of the complaints I hear from staff when a person is manic is "they act like staff". That is part of being grandiose. The opposite of feeling absolutely worthless in depression is feeling grandiose in mania. People with mania may believe that they are important persons of power. For many people with developmental disabilities, the perceived position of ultimate power is "staff". Hence, "he acts like he is staff.' Grandiosity may also present as "I'm going to college", or "I own McDonald's".

People with mania will frequently talk fast or sound pressured. If you have ever listened to Robin Williams do a comic monologue, you know what manic speech is. He goes from topic to topic to topic. I visualize pressured speech like someone shaking up a bottle of diet Pepsi then taking the top off. The liquid spray, or words, comes out fast and random. When a person is essentially non-verbal, like Ron, they may "sing song" non-stop or yell continuously.

Labile mood common in (mixed) mania often confuses the casual observer. The person may laugh too loud, suddenly cry, and then immediately roll off a litany of unprintable speech. These changes can all occur within 45 seconds, or altering moods may be present in one 24-hour period. The person is usually not cycling from –2 to +2 several times a day, but rather the extreme changes in mood are a variation of mood lability. The person may not necessarily experience internally all of these moods such as anger, sadness, or extreme happiness. They seem unable to hold onto any mood for any length of time. Mood lability is most commonly seen in mania, but at times may be seen in certain personality disorders.

At this stage of mania, a person may only sleep 4 – 6 hours. To monitor sleep, you may find it helpful, if not mandatory, to use the sleep chart (chart 4.4) found in the last chapter. Again, even though they may sleep very little, they will not be tired. You might begin to see weight loss because sitting down to eat is very difficult. Drive through food is too slow for them. These folks become so driven that they cannot slow down to focus on the mundane whether it is work, food, or sleep. Persons with mania cannot sit down to eat at the average group home table. You may only be able to get them to eat finger foods and beverages as they walk or run by. Indeed, if you try to get them to sit down to eat, you are inviting an act of aggression.

At a +3, the person with mania will have unlimited amounts of energy. I have seen people with full-blown mania go for over a week without sleep and not be tired. In the old days before medications, this non-stop activity would frequently be a cause of death since the body would literally exhaust itself. People with full mania can be very much out of control. They can also be very aggressive.

The good news about somebody who is manic and potentially aggressive is that they are also highly distractible. Betty could be ready to punch the daylights out of George. If I act fast, I can say, "Hey, Betty, come on and take a look at this what zit over here." Betty would probably investigate the what zit and momentarily forget pummeling George. The problem then becomes George, who doesn't forget, and starts to charge back after Betty. At that point, you need somebody to watch out for George.

To experience mania, the closest I can come is a kid-oriented pizza parlor where I occasionally have a lapse of sanity and take my girls. For the full effect, it is mandatory to go there on a rainy Saturday afternoon. Usually there are a minimum of 14 birthday parties going on with at least eight children per party. All 112 of the kids are screaming. In one corner of the restaurant, they have a bazillion tables and huge mechanical robots that sing these stupid songs about four decibels louder than anybody ever needs to hear them. In another corner, they have coin operated (coins purchased by doting grown-ups) video arcade and skeeball games with heavy balls (that's a wonderful thing to give small children who are hyped up—solid balls). All this game playing is in pursuit of tickets so that the children can exchange the tickets for a cheap plastic toy that will be lost in the car on the way home. In another corner they have mechanical rides that go up and down, side to side, and back and forth. Darlings with delicate stomachs then lose all the birthday cake, pizza, and caffeinated colas.

For true research of mania and mania relief, the place you want to stand is near the bathroom door. (Find something to do to look busy.) I have literally seen grandparents fight each other over the opportunity to take little Festus to the bathroom. The stimuli in this pleasure palace are so overwhelming that people will do almost anything to escape to the bathroom. I have watched women walk into the bathroom and heave a large sigh of relief at the silence. (Given all the diet pop I drink, I was originally there for traditional purposes, NOT weird research!)

As I gave this same example at an ARC conference, one woman raised her hand and said, "You know I used to work there." After I gave her my condolences, she went on to say, "I used to fight for the opportunity to clean the toilets, just to get out of the mayhem in the other room." Now I don't know about you, but I find it a sad state of affairs when you are fighting someone else for an opportunity to clean a toilet. For a person who is manic, living in the average group home or attending the average day program is like taking up permanent residence in that pizza parlor without a bathroom pass.

Like the grandparents fighting in the pizza place, I have seen people with mania deliberately start a fight just to get to the "time-out room". Sometimes a person with a disability recognizes that he is stressed out, but they are not allowed the normal releases you and I enjoy. When you and I are stressed out at work, we may turn on the computer for a quick game of solitaire. We may wander down the hallway to talk to a coworker. It may be time to investigate the pop machine or see if some other department has free food setting out. When all else fails, there is always lunchtime.

Unfortunately, many of the people that we work with are not allowed time outs on their schedule, only on ours. Perhaps we could begin to use a quiet corner as a reward as opposed to punishment. Let the person who is stressed out go to the quiet area BEFORE she hits someone. This is therapy, not punishment. (And remember, we are not allowed to call four point leather restraints on a gurney a therapeutic moment. Necessary perhaps, but not a therapeutic moment.)

Depression and bipolar disorder are lumped together historically because they both involve changes in mood. Unlike depression where we at least have some understanding that serotonin and perhaps norepinephrine are involved in the symptoms, the actual nervous system deficits involved in bipolar disorder are still to a great extent uncertain. Since mania is the opposite of depression, wouldn't it be easy, if mania were brought on by an increase in serotonin? Although serotonin is involved in mania, there is much more to the puzzle.

Researchers are exploring the theory that there is a flood of many of the neurotransmitters going from one nerve cell to the other. Over-excitement of neurotransmitters is suspected, but the exact understanding, however, of which neurotransmitters and how and why it happens is still under investigation. We do know that there is a familial tendency and genetic component to bipolar disorder. It is common to see people with bipolar disorder having either a history of alcoholism, bipolar disorder, or major depression in their families. Consequently, although we have several medications that work well to treat bipolar disorder much of the time, we are still not certain exactly how or why they work.

Lithium carbonate (commonly abbreviated LiCO3) has been the drug of choice, if not the only choice, for people with bipolar disorder for many decades. Although it certainly helped many people, some people simply didn't respond sufficiently or were unable to tolerate lithium. Practitioners then tried to supplement with older antipsychotics, Valium type medicines, blood pressure medicines, ECT, antidepressants, and anything else they thought might help.

In the search, several other medications found useful for treatment of bipolar disorder actually came out of treatments for epilepsy or seizure disorder. These are valproic acid/divalproex (Depakene, Depakote), carbamazepine (Tegretol, Carbatrol – extended release form of carbamazepine), oxcarbazepine (Trileptal – similar to carbamazepine, but not blood level dependent), gabapentin (Neurontin), lamotrigine (Lamictal), and topiramate (Topamax). (Chart 5.2) Of these, only Depakote, as of this writing, has FDA approval for use in mania in bipolar disorder. Lamictal was recently approved for maintenance therapy of bipolar disorder. This means that the makers of Depakote and Lamictal can include bipolar disorder as a reason to use it in their information package about the medicine. Since the other medications are FDA approved for other purposes, it is permissible to use them for reasons other than seizure control, but it is referred to as "off-label" usage.

Besides the seizure medications and lithium, the most promising treatment options for both phases of bipolar disorder are the new "atypical" antipsychotics discussed in chapter 7. These newer drugs have been useful in ways beyond typical understanding of the older antipsychotics. This is likely due to their effects on multiple neurotransmitters in the brain. At this time, only Zyprexa, Risperidol and Seroquel have FDA approval for use in mania (although others are in the process of research trials for FDA approval). Clinically, however, the others have also shown promise. Other medication options include thyroid medicines, Valium type drugs, and calcium channel blockers normally used for cardiac purposes.

Approximately ten to twelve years ago, practitioners would give the person who was aggressive carbamazepine (Tegretol). The idea was "we don't know why, but Tegretol sometimes stopped aggression." The reason Tegretol worked in many of these cases is that Tegretol is often effective in treating bipolar disorder. Therefore when someone is aggressive as a result of mood instability, Tegretol, Depakote and the others often work. In addition, all the above antiseizure medicines have been useful in irritability associated with other brain disturbances such as closed head injuries.

People with developmental disabilities have a higher than average chance of also having a seizure disorder. In part, it was the recognition that some people with seizures and bipolar disorder suddenly got better when we changed their seizure medicines from the older medications such as phenytoin (Dilantin) and phenobarbital to one of the newer agents that led to our current treatment approaches. Since Depakote and Tegretol (both of which are also available in extended release formats for ease of taking, and hopefully fewer side effects) are still primarily used for seizures, it is optimal to work with a neurologist to see if either Tegretol or Depakote (or Neurontin, Lamictal, or Topamax if necessary) would work for the seizure disorder as well when the person has both disorders. These medications are NOT interchangeable. They each have unique properties in terms of seizure control (work for some types of seizures, but not others), and whether they work best for depression, mania, or both.

Julia was a wonderful woman who lived in her own home with support. Her supporters clearly love her, but they are worn out. She is busy all the time, but has trouble finishing anything. She talks non-stop. Staff wondered if she had some type of anxiety disorder. Coincidentally, however, when anti-anxiety medicines were given for dental appointments, she seemed to get worse. The neighbors were complaining that Julia was up at all hours of the night. She never seemed tired. The only other medication that Julia was on was Depakote for a seizure disorder.

As you can see from Chart 5.2, the normal blood range for Depakote is 50 to 100 ug/ml (some say as high as 125, or even 150, but then the risk of side effects is greater). Julia's blood level was 52.6 12 hours after last dose. Since she had been seizure free for years, no one thought there was any need to increase her dosage. I met with her primary care doctor who was prescribing the Depakote.

Medications For Use In Bipolar Disorder (Manic - Depression)
Chart 5.2

First Line Choices	Recommended Drug Range	Potential Toxic Range
carbamazepine (Tegretol, Tegretol XR) (not FDA indicated)	6 - 12 mcg/ml	>15 mcg/ml
lithium carbonate (Lithium, Eskalith CR, Lithobid)	0.5 - 1.2 mEq/L	>1.5 mEq/L
Olanzapine/Zyprexa	10 - 15mg/day	N.A.
valproic acid (Depakote, Depakene)	50 - 125 μg/ml	>150μg/ml

(Risperidol and Seroquel are, and most newer atypicals will be, FDA approved for mania or bipolar soon. See Chapter 7.)

2nd Line/Augmentation	Other Options
gabapentin (Neurontin) lamotrigine (Lamictal)[1] topiramate (Topamax)[2] oxcarbatepine (Trileptal)	ECT Atypical Antipsychotics Thyroid Replacement Valium-type Medication Calcium Channel Blockers, i.e., Amlodipine

[1] Must start dosage low and go very slow to avoid potentially life threatening rash. Use half dosage if given with valproic acid. Double dose if used with carbamazepine. Recently released by the FDA for maintenance therapy.

[2] Cognitive difficulties common when started. May help to prevent other medication related weight gain.

The doctor wanted to help with Julia's more difficult behaviors, but wasn't sure how. Given the lack of need for sleep, constant activity and talking, a preliminary diagnosis of hypomania (lower level mania symptoms without known periods of depression – a variation of bipolar disorder) seemed appropriate. She may have even had full bipolar disorder, partially treated. As she was already on Depakote, the easiest move was to increase the dosage, and thus blood level. The last I heard, people commented that she comes home from work tired like everyone else and really seems to enjoy her life even more. Even the neighbors are reported to be resting better.

As long as we are discussing seizure medicines, phenytoin and phenobarbital have been around for a long time. Both are relatively cheap when it comes to seizure control. A day's supply of phenobarbital will only cost a bit of pocket change. A day's supply of Lamictal, however, will require several pieces of green paper with pictures of dead presidents (or several round coins with swimming birds on them for those of you north of the boarder.)! Price per pill economics aside, however, research has shown that phenobarbital and Mysoline (a phenobarbital cousin) can cause agitation/aggression all on their own without any other psychiatric symptomatology.

My first recommendation when asked to evaluate a person who is aggressive and on phenobarbital or Mysoline for seizure control, is to request the prescribing doctor to consider changing to a different seizure medication. Every person that I have seen switched has had a marked decrease in aggression without any other treatment. This is another of those examples as discussed in the beginning of the book demonstrating that we must never stop looking at the whole picture...especially physical needs first.

As with many with bipolar disorder, it seems that for folks with developmental disabilities, lithium carbonate as a single agent has been less than effective. I believe that the primary reason for this goes back to the root cause of many disorders in persons with disabilities. That is, the brain has malfunctions. Because Depakote and Tegretol were derived more for neurological purposes, it may be that they have a better impact on the brain than the lithium carbonate could account for, but this is unknown territory at this time. In the last several years, I have seen more prescribers use Valproic acid/divalproex (Depakote) as the drug of choice for the treatment of bipolar disorder with or without a developmental disability. This is also suggested by research from N.I.H. (Post, 2000). Lamictal, Trileptal, Neurontin, and Topamax (which are NOT currently monitored by blood level tests) have been used as adjunct medications, which are added on when the primary medication doesn't seem to be providing enough relief for the individual symptomatology, but not as primary medications for treatment of bipolar disorder.

Side effects of the big three medications, that is Lithium, Depakote, and Tegretol, and the toxic effects of these medications are not the same. Side effects most frequently occur when the medications are begun or increased. All of these medications can cause slowing of mental processes and caution should be used when starting any medication. A decision must be made on whether the disorder being treated or the side effects of the treatment are most harmful to the person. Other side effects of lithium include thirst, increased urination (because it interferes with water recovery in the kidneys), intolerance to heat, mild tremor, and allergic rash. A long-term side effect of lithium is hypothyroidism. Side effects of Depakote and Tegretol may include cognitive impairment, GI upset, pancreas, liver and/or blood irregularities, allergic rash, tremor, sluggishness, and lethargy. Weight gain, hair loss, and ovarian irregularities may be also seen with Depakote.

Lithium, Depakote, and Tegretol are all blood level dependent. That means, for a person to achieve maximum helpful effects without harmful toxic effects, several blood tests must be performed. The blood level of the medication must also be correlated to the person's clinical picture. One person may only need 300 mg of lithium at night to obtain a blood level of 0.6 and be relatively symptom free. The next person may require 600 mg of lithium carbonate three times a day to obtain a blood level of 0.6 and be still experiencing symptoms. This helps us understand why people may need more than one mood stabilizer.

Toxic effects of Lithium, Tegretol, and Depakote may literally look as if the person were drunk. The person may experience irregular gait. He may be very difficult to arouse or his speech may become very, very garbled. He may complain of feeling really lousy, like he has a hangover. In another lesson of Sue's "DD" Handbook, a person will only become toxic on these medications on a Friday evening before a holiday weekend when nobody can be reached. On Tuesday morning when anybody can be reached, no one ever seems to become toxic.

Any caregiver who is associated with the person on most seizure medications or lithium, should always be aware that if the person is acting unusually tired, stumbling with slurred speech or difficult to arouse, DO NOT give the next dosage of medication. You can do more harm by giving it than by withholding it when the person is not toxic. The person with suspected toxicity will need an emergency blood draw at their usual laboratory or at the closest emergency room. When a person is toxic, medications will probably be held for a few days and either reduced or gradually resumed. If the blood levels for these medications reach toxic levels, they may cause very serious damage to the liver and/or kidneys, even to the point of death.

I am sure all of you with inquiring minds wonder what kinds of things can cause a person to become toxic on their medications. Toxicity from Lithium, Depakote, or Tegretol occurs when the concentration levels of the drug increase in the body. If a person has diarrhea, vomiting or is sweating excessively, the person is at risk for dehydration. As the internal fluid levels in the body decrease, the concentration of medication in the blood increases. A person with the flu virus, for example, is in danger of becoming toxic. A person placed on a diuretic (water pill for high blood pressure or edema) could become toxic very quickly.

Lithium toxicity is less likely to occur from medication combinations other than perhaps ibuprofen. Lithium is a salt that initially will make people thirstier. Table salt is generally not restricted for a person taking lithium. If a fluid restriction is necessary for other reasons, the person should be carefully monitored. Generally it doesn't matter how much liquid a person usually drinks per day (a little or a lot – within reason) as long as the amount stays reasonably constant each day.

Carbamazepine/Tegretol toxicity may occur because it activates the liver. That is, it causes the liver to work harder. When the liver works harder, it metabolizes or chews up the carbamazepine and other medications faster. As the dosage is increased, the liver works harder and chews up more Tegretol. At some point, this chewing up and activating cross over in a person who was having difficulty reaching a therapeutic level. The next small increase at this "crossover" point may suddenly cause toxicity.

In addition to this, Tegretol goes through one of the major garbage disposal ports in the liver. When other medications need to go through this same port, it can cause either levels of Tegretol to increase, or levels of the other medication to increase. For example, Tegretol causes oral contraceptives to be chewed up faster than anticipated. Women taking oral contraceptives could become pregnant if they are also taking Tegretol. Medications that may slow the chewing up of Tegretol thus increasing the level include Erythromycin type antibiotics such as Biaxin.

I have seen people who have been prescribed Biaxin while also on Tegretol become toxic on their Tegretol within a matter of 24 hours or less. INH used for treatment of tuberculosis can also increase Tegretol levels. Trileptal is a cousin of carbamazepine that is similar in design and properties, but is not blood level dependent nor is it involved in the same garbage disposal pathway.

Before starting Lithium, Depakote, or Tegretol, individuals should undergo some preliminary health screens. The person should have had a thorough physical recently. Initial lab tests should include a complete blood count, liver and kidney function tests, and a urinalysis. With lithium, an evaluation of thyroid function is also necessary, and an EKG is recommended for anyone over the age of 40. Blood levels and appropriate other screens should be done every seven to ten days after each dosage change. When the person has reached a satisfactory blood level and is psychiatrically stable, blood levels have been recommended as well as liver and kidney function tests for Depakote every 3 months. (Clinicians are also noting elevated ammonia levels secondary to valproic acid that may result in behavioral disturbances.) Some labs suggest every 6 months to one year, but our state recommends every 3...check with your local authorities. For Tegretol, a complete (or partial) blood count as well as perhaps hepatic function should also be done every three months (see note on frequency above). Full laboratory tests are recommended yearly while on these medicines. The blood levels of the medicine are generally drawn 10 to 12 hours after the last dosage (please talk to your doctor if using an extended release format of these medications.). Usually the morning dose is held until the blood is taken. If the blood is taken soon after the medication is given it may not give an accurate level. Trileptol and Tegretol can both decrease sodium levels.

When I first met Terri, she reminded me of some wild untamed creature. She screamed almost non-stop. She appeared to deliberately fall if given the chance. She violently assaulted people. She had few apparent skills, and no friends.

The last time I saw her, we looked through books together. She had recently had her hair done. I am told that she informed the stylist that she was not satisfied with the first style, and for the stylist to try again. She looked very sharp. I had been covering for her primary psychiatrist who was out on leave, and I always explain that I am a nurse practitioner. She asked me where her doctor was. You must understand that Terri was said to be profoundly retarded and until recently, few of us knew she could talk. Before I could explain where the doctor was, staff interrupted and tried to tell Terri that I was the doctor. Terri very slowly explained to them (so that hopefully they would understand with only one explanation!) "No! That's Sue. Where's the doctor?"

Terry's psychiatrist (the one who had been on leave) had been slowly reducing the Mellaril that Terri had been on for many, many years and placed her on Depakote. The Depakote is controlling the bipolar disorder that she probably suffered from for years. The removal of the clouding effects of the older antipsychotic allowed her wonderful personality complete with the wicked sense of humor to emerge.

When I had my last sinus infection, frankly, the 14-day course of antibiotics took me 16.5 days to complete. I had trouble always remembering to take them. In addition, once I felt better (about day 5), it's hard to convince myself to keep taking medicine...even though I KNOW the importance of finishing the entire prescription. I think most people do not like taking medications when they feel fine. In chronic illnesses such as depression and bipolar disorder, this may not be an option.

Even a few years ago, when a person was treated for one of these disorders, we would recommend 6 to 12 months of medications. If the person continued to do well, we would consider tapering or discontinuing the medicine. In part this was because many older medications had some nasty side effects.

What we have discovered, especially with bipolar disorder, is that many if not most people would experience a severe reoccurrence of the illness. In addition, the medicine they responded well to the first time might not work as well, if at all, the second time around. In bipolar disorder, the risk of suicide increases dramatically when the individual is no longer taking appropriate medication. For these reasons, practitioners are often reluctant to stop these medications except in the presence of serious side effects or strong desire to quit on the part of the individual. In general, the sooner a person relapses, the more likely they will require treatment for life.

This practice of maintaining people on medications after symptoms have been relieved flies in the face of older regulations that view use of psychiatric medications in persons with disabilities as "behavior control." In days gone by, if a person was doing well, i.e., not aggressive, their medications had to be reduced or the system would face penalties from regulatory agencies. This is logical if one is talking of chemical restraint. When treating a psychiatric illness, however, this automatic reduction plan is nonsense. If my blood sugars are normalized by daily taking 36 units of insulin, I will not "reward" myself for good blood glucose levels, by dropping my insulin to 27 units (25% reduction). Antibiotics will eliminate or cure a sinus infection. Psychiatric medications such as lithium treat the symptoms, but do not cure the illness, anymore than insulin "cures" diabetes.

When I first met Cindy, I had to wait while she changed clothes 5 times. She was hyperverbal, intrusive, and hadn't slept for 36 hours. She was treated "behaviorally" for aggression for years, and received increasing and decreasing dosages of Lithium. It was increased when she was doing poorly, and decreased every time she was doing well. It took years for her to leave the institution. She also had mild mental retardation, and so for years was thought that she couldn't have bipolar disorder. Once placed in the community, our psychiatrist added

Depakote, and maintained both dosages of Depakote and Lithium. The good times lasted longer and longer. Unfortunately, Cindy felt that she was unjustly being punished because she viewed being "good" (not manic), as a sign that she shouldn't have to take medications. She died recently for reasons unrelated to her bipolar illness, but never understood that her doctor was giving her the best care possible.

Chapter 6

Anxiety: It's A Panic

Psalms 23:4
Even though I walk through the valley of the shadow of
death, I will fear no evil, for You are with me.

I remember very vividly my first panic attack, even though as a 17-year old in high school, anxiety was already a common phenomenon. Some days that zit would pop right out on the end of my nose. Why did it have to pop out on the day that I shared math class with the cutest guy in 11th grade? Other sources of anxiety included tolerating the hot lunches in the cafeteria, and most particularly, riding the school bus. If I were really lucky, my older brother would drop me off at school on his way in to work. Somehow riding home on the bus didn't seem as bad, but riding it in the morning was more than a 17-year old should ever tolerate (I'll have to rethink this now that I have a high-schooler!).

The day came that my brother was unable to drive me to school. But wait . . . I had a driver's license now! I coaxed and pleaded with my dad to let me use his car. He and mom were driving into work together anyway so that extra car was just sitting there in the driveway. I would be careful. Dad spoke forever about the hazards of possible slick spots on a cold morning, but I heard almost none of that. I knew when he began warning me about the slick spots that the battle had been won and the car keys would soon be mine. "The Talk" and scrambling to get all of my stuff together before school caused me to be just a few minutes late. I decided to pick up some time on the one long stretch up to the high school. That's when it happened.

Just as the speedometer hit 50 in a 35 MPH zone, I hit a patch of black ice. My dad's car did a complete 360-degree "donut" and was on its way around for another turn when the back end headed towards the ditch. My entire 17 years flashed before my eyes. Since there weren't any cars around, I wasn't particularly worried about my own mortality. The anxiety was caused from KNOW-ING I would have to face my father when his car was completely smashed in the ditch. There wasn't enough time just then for prayer, but God must have heard me anyway. The back tires of the car drove right into somebody's unknown driveway and stopped. There was not a scratch, a mark, or even a tire out of alignment on the car, but I was a wreck.

My heart was beating out of control, and my legs felt like Jell-O left out on an August day. My hands were shaking, and I needed to go back home for a clean shirt because the sweat stains and the smells were more than I could tolerate. Besides that, the stomach upset and instant flight of diarrhea let me know that the flu or some such terrible thing had just hit me. Actually no flu bug hit me; I had simply had an over-run of stress hormones.

What I had experienced on that slick winter day was a rush of anxiety. To some extent, this anxious stress reaction is a protective mechanism. Back in the days of the dinosaurs, Ogg looked at the dinosaur and decided to retreat fast to avoid being the dinosaur's supper, or run like heck to catch the dinosaur for his supper. This is referred to as the "fight or flight syndrome". The stress response, for both positive and negative stress, begins with cortisol being released from the brain and prepares the body to react and respond. Thus, Ogg had the energy to run or fight, and this reaction continues to work for us today.

When I lecture, I conduct my own unofficial research study. If I announce that you have a significant report due in one month's time which your grade or job relies upon, you will most likely respond in one of the following ways. A certain percentage of you would set down this book right now and rush off to start that report. In fact, the anxiety is probably already cooking for a few of you as you begin to contemplate, "Oh my gosh is there a report out there that I might need to be working on?"

There will be another larger percentage of you who will gradually begin to chip away at the project and be reasonably close to completion at month's end. There is another possibly even larger chunk of you who wait until the night before the project is due to get started. When I ask the reason for waiting until the night before to get the project done, the universal response is "I work best under pressure." The sluggards who wait until the night before are to some extent correct. They get enough of an adrenaline boost to get them motivated to get the project done. For those people in the first group who started it the first day that they heard about the project, just thinking about waiting until the night before the project is due is enough to send them into a cold sweat.

When we are unable to tolerate stress reactions, we often have symptoms suggestive of an anxiety disorder. Clearly, we must differentiate between the people who are in crisis versus a long-term anxiety disorder. Any of us may feel anxious in a crisis situation. Indeed, attempting to treat momentary crisis reactions with medications may impair positive coping and growth. When those feelings of anxiety go beyond the crisis or occur when no real stress is even around, however, there may be reason for concern.

Most anxiety disorders have longer time criteria, i.e., symptoms lasting longer than 6 months, or a point of recognizing that the fear is excessive by usual standards. Anxiety disorders are very closely associated with the depressive disorders. In fact, there is approximately a

60% overlap between depression and anxiety (That is, symptoms of both anxiety AND depression occur at the same time in those 60%.). Just as depression and bi-polar disorder are frequently found in persons with disabilities, anxiety disorders are also commonly present.

Among my many quirks is the ability to recall my addresses and phone numbers from when I was a kid up to the present time. I can recall other vague, useless pieces of information including the best sale price of peanut butter at any given store ($0.99 for the store brand, 18-oz. Size, $1.27 for the name brand stuff). I remember whether or not the coupon that could be doubled in my coupon holder would create a better price than the current detergent price I am looking at in the warehouse club. You would think with such brain cells I would never have difficulty recalling things.

Wrong, my problem is names. I will be talking with someone I know well and for the life of me I cannot recall the person's name. (This really annoys the daylights out of my children too when I call them by the dog's name.) Whenever it happens, which is quite often, I get that little pit in my stomach that tells me, "Oh no, here I go again, I can't recall this person's name and I know I know it."

While my name-recall handicap is embarrassing, Roger's quest for names as well as the person's car type has a tendency to get him into trouble. Roger is a 27-year old man with autism. Given the anxiety that he has in trying to straighten and organize his world, he feels it necessary to know everyone's last name as well as the type of car they drive. It's not that he would actually ever do anything with this information such as look it up on the web and try and ruin your credit rating, he simply NEEDS to know this information. Unfortunately 20-year old young ladies in the mall don't want to pass this information on when approached by a stranger. When they don't give him this information, Roger takes it as a personal threat to his own safety. He then becomes agitated, has been known to flap his arms, bite his hands and start to flay around. He has not actually hurt anyone else, but he has scared others. Roger wanted a job in a fast food restaurant. Every time he got around all those strangers, however, he HAD to ask their name and car type. This roadblock to employment prompted the referral to our clinic.

I noticed in our initial meeting together that Roger had a series of questions that he asked his mother. His mother responded with the same answers that she has been repeating for the last twenty some years. The assurance of the same answers quickly calmed him and he was able to sit through the entire meeting. When Roger asked when the meeting would be over, I gave him a time on the clock without really thinking about it. With luck, and dawning realization, I was able to come within about 45 seconds of my designated time of ending the meeting. Roger was extremely relieved. As I realized the situation I had set myself up in, I am afraid I would have had to end the meeting around that time regardless of whether or not I was finished because Roger was.

As with the affective disorders, there are many theories for the origin of anxiety disorders. It could have been some misconfiguration or structural defect in the brain. Most of the current work is looking at the HPA axis (hypothalamus-pituitary-adrenal gland) portion of the brain due to its control of cortisol and ultimately adrenaline. Severe stress in childhood may also alter developing portions of the brain increasing the likelihood of anxiety disorders. Given the success rates of the SSRI's in treating anxiety, some researchers suggest that there is another serotonin connection, and misfires here create anxiety symptoms. It could be that your body's response is over sensitive to even normal amounts of stress hormones (i.e., adrenaline) that cruise through your blood vessels. Again, there appears to be a familial component to anxiety disorders. Additionally, some people do not gain adequate coping strategies to deal with life's stresses. The theories behind anxiety disorders continue to be explored. Since there are different types of anxiety problems, it makes sense that there could be more than one cause and more than one treatment.

Jenna worried all the time. If the bus was late in coming, she worried that there had been an accident. If work was limited at the day program, she wondered if there would ever be work again. When it was time for her physical, she usually threw up beforehand thinking she might be dying. Her mom could occasionally calm her down with a lot of reassurance, but not always. Jenna understood that her concerns were extreme, yet she couldn't stop worrying any more than she could stop breathing.

Albert stood in the corner of his new group home. Rather than facing the corner as someone with depression might, Al stood with his back to the corner. He seemed to need to know where everyone in the home was at all times. Since several others in Al's home were hearing impaired, staff had become accustom to gently tapping folks on the shoulder to get their attention. The first time someone tapped Al, he almost leaped out of his skin. Albert and Jenna both suffered from anxiety disorders.

Symptoms of Generalized Anxiety Disorder, GAD, (DSM IV-TR)

A. Excessive anxiety and worry lasting more than six months.

B. Person finds it difficult to control the worry.

C. Anxiety and worry associated with at least three of the following:
- Restlessness, keyed-up, or "on edge."
- Easily fatigued.
- Difficulty concentrating, mind goes blank.
- Irritability.
- Muscle tension.
- Sleep disturbances.

Chart 6.1

GAD Generalized Anxiety Disorder (Chart 6.1) involves excessive worry like Jenna's lasting at least 6 months about a number of events. The person finds it hard to control the worry. She may experience many of the symptoms of panic (Chart 6.2), The person may be very restless or on hyper-alert at all times. These people know where everyone in the environment is. They are the ones who stand in the corner. Like Al, folks with anxiety may have their back to the corner so that they can watch where everyone is at any and all times. While I may still feel anxious on icy roads, a person with GAD may feel these symptoms for much of their waking and attempted sleeping life.

In most anxiety disorders there are many of the common symptoms of panic or severe anxiety (Chart 6.2). In GAD, since symptoms are often physical, people frequently see their medical doctors many times before an anxiety disorder is identified. In fact, current research suggests that people will undergo many, many medical tests for many years before psychiatric treatment is sought. It is important, however, to rule out the medical disorders first before assuming that the person has an anxiety disorder. Just to complicate things, the person may have an anxiety disorder AND other medical complications such as high blood pressure or ulcers, perhaps as a result of long term anxiety.

Chart 6.2

Panic/Anxiety Symptoms, DSM-IV-TR
(Not the same as Panic Disorder)

A period of intense fear in which four or more of the following start suddenly and reach a peak within 10 minutes.

1. Heart palpitations, racing or pounding heart.
2. Sweating.
3. Shaking or trembling.
4. Shortness of breath.
5. Choking sensation.
6. Chest pain.
7. GI upset.
8. Dizziness, lightheadedness or faint.
9. Feel like the experience or you are "unreal."
10. Fear of "going crazy."
11. Fear of dying.
12. Numbness or tingling in arms and/or legs.
13. Chills or hot flashes.

See DSM IV-TR for "panic disorder."

Dave told me I could tell his story regarding obsessive-compulsive disorder (OCD- Chart 6.3). A few years ago, Dave's group home manager asked me casually if clomipramine (Anafranil) could cause constipation.

Thinking it was only a simple question and it was five minutes to five on Friday afternoon, I answered, "Yes" and turned to leave. As I was about to walk out the door, I noticed the look on her face. She then said, "I am not sure if I should mention this . . .?" I always love those opening lines.

She went on to say that Dave had been very constipated lately. Feeling like I was about to be taken by a joke I asked, "How constipated?" "Well . . . We gave him some magnesium citrate." Mag citrate is that stuff that comes in a little green bottle and they try and convince you it tastes like 7Up. It doesn't. One bottle, however, is usually enough to clean the average person out for intestinal x-rays. If Dave required a bottle of mag citrate, I knew that he had been very constipated. I started getting concerned even though it was now 4:57 on a Friday afternoon. How much mag citrate did he require? (Hoping that perhaps it was only a half a bottle) She then hemmed, hawed and looked a little sheepish.

I honestly don't know where they got the medical order for the following dosage of medication. It was one of those situations where I really just didn't want to know the answer. "SIX!!?" Staff gave Dave six bottles of magnesium citrate on the previous Saturday morning. As if this wasn't bad enough, he did not explode until Monday afternoon. Unfortunately for Dave, most medication information sheets include constipation, and nobody had really paid attention to the fact that Anafranil could be constipating. Even at 5:02 on a Friday afternoon, something had to be done.

Dave has Down syndrome. He had been labeled "non-compliant" for years. His violence prompted his home staff to approach the psychiatrist. He became very violent if anyone sat in his chair. In fact if anyone sat in a seat other than his or her usual chair, Dave became upset. He could only leave his day program at 3:00 p.m. If he had an appointment and had to leave five minutes early, he became easily agitated. If the van was five minutes late, he threw things. He was so insistent on sameness that he never seemed to be able to enjoy anything. He rarely spoke. He certainly didn't smile.

Dave's psychiatrist diagnosed his "non-compliant behavior" as obsessive-compulsive disorder. Although the Anafranil (first medication identified to help with OCD) helped, he still had problems. Attempts to increase his medicine resulted in the now-realized constipation. Dave's team asked if anything else could be done. Although this was the early 90's, it was already known that fluoxetine (Prozac) helped to treat OCD.

At our last meeting, Dave told me about his recent trip to Florida. He flew down alone to visit his parents who are now retired in the "Mickey Mouse" part of Florida. He has a job at a local hamburger establishment where he works five days a week. He takes independent transportation to and from work. He continues to do quite well.

In addition to compulsive, ritualistic behaviors, many people with OCD experience recurring, intrusive, disturbing thoughts that they know are of their own making. OCD can be diagnosed if either obsessions, compulsions OR both are present. Since many persons with disabilities have trouble with communication, obsessions are harder to assess, but it can be done. Most people with obsessions know the ideas, images, and fears are not real. In spite of this, they cannot stop the thoughts. Often the obsessions are of perceived unpleasant subjects such as unusual sexual activities, or dislike for another person. Some people attempt to deal with these thoughts through repetitive actions such as washing their hands 23 times before eating. Some people insist on absolute sameness in routines, staff, and activities, such that change in routine is felt to be catastrophic.

Besides the DSM-IV-TR, (Chart 6.3) another useful screening device is the compulsive behavior checklist designed for persons with developmental disabilities (Gedye, 1992). Support staff can complete this scale in a short period of time, yet it still provides comprehensive data for accurate diagnosing.

Persons with autism or pervasive development disorders frequently suffer from difficulties in dealing with change in their routine. Whether a person with autism can also be diagnosed with obsessive -compulsive disorder (or OCD) is sometimes dependent upon how well they match the criteria for OCD in the DSM-IV-TR and sometimes according to practitioner's discretion.

Symptoms of Obsessive-Compulsive Disorder, OCD (DSM IV-TR)

Obsessions and/or compulsions present.

Obsessions (all four criteria):
- Recurrent, persistant thoughts that are intrusive, inappropriate, and cause marked anxiety or distress.
- Thoughts suggested above are not worries about real-life problems.
- Person attempts to ignore, suppress thoughts, or to neutralize them with other thoughts or actions.
- Person recognizes thoughts are of his own making.

Compulsions (both criteria):
- Repetative behaviors in response to obsessions *or* according to rigidly held rules.
- Behaviors are aimed at reducing or preventing distress.

Additionally, obsessions or compulsions take up more than 1 hour per day or significantly impair social, relational, or occupational funcioning.

Chart 6.3

Shirley was a lady I got to know who had one of the most unusual introductory sheets that I had ever seen. According to the request for services form that I had received, Shirley (who had autism) was experiencing "deliberate incontinence". She never seemed able to get to the bathroom on time although repeated medical tests revealed nothing.

I got lucky on this one. The van for Shirley's group home broke down. Since time was of the essence, I was asked to see her and her team at her home. That broken van taught me a valuable lesson. Whenever possible, I now try to see the person in their usual setting(s), i.e., home or work site. On this day, I noticed that the kitchen was between Shirley and the bathroom. Once she had the urge to use the bathroom, she would have to go through the kitchen. On her way through the kitchen, I watched her straighten the soap dish (three times), and make sure the cupboard doors were all closed (after having opened and closed them each three times). She also had to make sure that the trashcan was at the right angle, again three times. She rehung the washcloth hanging over the sink three times. Once she finished all this and checked it all over one more time, she had a toiletting accident as she entered the bathroom. When staff tried to move her towards the bathroom faster and cut her routine short, she would bite herself, and start over at the beginning.

Imagine, if you will, continuous fearful thoughts going through your head or at the very least feeling that the world may come to an end if all your socks are not sorted exactly by color and thread type. Persons with OCD attempt to deal with internal stress by making sure that the external world remains consistent. To some extent, we all experience OCD moments. Let's be honest here, how many of you have ever turned someone's toilet paper around because they had it going "the wrong way"? Have you ever fought over where you squeeze the toothpaste? Many new couples have their first big fight when the holidays arrive. "BUT D.E.A.R...We always open presents on Christmas Eve!" We all develop habits or traditions that are hard to change, but when our very core self is threatened by the thought of change, there are problems.

Sometimes our worries almost have a reason for being. Have you ever had an important interview for which you had to get up at 6:00 AM? You lie down in bed and begin to wonder, "Did I set the alarm clock?" You get up, check the alarm clock and lie back down. Upon lying down, you stop to think, "Now, when I checked it, did I turn the alarm clock on or turn it off?" You get back up, check the alarm clock one last time and lie back down again. At this point you remember that you have to take a copy of your resume to the appointment. You get up to make sure you have that by your briefcase ready to head out the door the next morning. After checking all these things six or seven times you may finally be able to lie down but you are certainly unable to fall right to sleep. At least, I couldn't!

While many of us may experience some of these briefly, for people with OCD, these thoughts and behaviors can take over their entire day and life. Some people can literally not make it out the door to work because of the hours it requires to check and recheck situations. Some people may spend several hours in the shower not actually showering but checking and rechecking that a certain body part is washed sufficiently and creating sores in the process.

Recently I saw a gentleman that I had been seeing for "intermittent explosive disorder" for several years. He had been diagnosed at another clinic and came to us on a very regulated antipsychotic medication. He and his family were very resistive to ever changing it so he tolerated the biweekly blood draws that went with his medication. On this particular occasion, I noted that his hands looked very red and had many sores on them. When I mentioned the sores on his hands, he commented that he wasn't surprised because he had been cleaning his apartment with bleach. Wondering if he had mismeasured the amount of bleach in the washing solution, I asked more questions. He assured me that he was using the accurate bleach solution, but that he was going through over a gallon of bleach a week! I couldn't understand why this should be since he has a small studio apartment.

He was using the bleach solution to completely wash his apartment (walls, counters, doors, windows, etc.) three times a day—every day. He had heard that there was going to be an inspection from the group home management regarding his semi-independent living situation. Out of fear of losing his living arrangement, it spun him into the need to clean on such a compulsive basis. We also began to question several other areas and realized that some of his "intermittent explosions" had OCD qualities to them. He was started on Celexa and within four months he was significantly better.

Like Shirley, some people with OCD attempt to maintain personal control (over anxiety) by constantly arranging things and checking them. When other people attempt to stop them from arranging, or make changes in the routine, the person with OCD may respond by attacking herself or the changer. The changer is seen as interrupting the only way that she knows to cope. An individual's aggression, while regrettable, is understandable. If you absolutely knew that washing your hands would save you from catastrophic illness, what would you do to someone who tried to stop you? The answer lies in helping the person find better ways to cope with stress. Here the answer lies partly with medications and partly by teaching them new ways to control their reactions to the environment.

Many people with OCD can be assisted to control their impulses with behavioral techniques found in cognitive behavioral therapy. Medications may also be a valuable tool in the treatment of OCD by producing a drop in symptoms (but usually not complete absence). The best response is seen when both therapies are used together. The most common medications used for the treatment of OCD today are Clomipramine (Anafranil) and the SSRI's including Prozac, Zoloft, Paxil, Luvox, Celexa, and Lexapro. Although officially classified as antidepressants, the SSRI's as a group have been shown to be very effective in all of the anxiety disorders. These medications have also been shown effective for the ritualistic behaviors associated with autism. (Since persons with autism may experience a higher than usual rate of bipolar disorder, caution must be taken that the SSRI's do not unveil an underlying cycling mood disorder.) Also, when used for OCD, the SSRI's may take up to 3 months before they begin to show a response.

Posttraumatic stress disorder (PTSD) (Chart 6.4) is unfortunately all too common in persons with developmental disabilities. The reason for this is simple. They have been subjected to incredible amounts of abuse and neglect. Some experts estimate that the percentage of physical or sexual abuse in adult men who have been institutionalized to be 60%! The estimates for institutionalized women are even higher at 80%! Dr. Ruth Ryan (1993) found that approximately 16% of persons with a history of abuse (regardless of where it occurred or by whom) also have PTSD. The simple math says that far too many currently or previously institutionalized adults that have experienced abuse will show signs of trauma. Although all persons who have been subjected to abuse will show some signs of the trauma, the full criteria of PTSD must be met in order for the diagnosis to be made. Often problem behaviors go uninvestigated and without the understanding of the damage that such abuse can create, too

---

Symptoms of Post Traumatic Stress Disorder, PTSD (DSM IV-TR)

Experienced, witnessed or confronted severe threat of death or injury AND responded to the above with intense fear, helplessness, or horror. Traumatic event is re-experienced by at least one of the following:
- Intrusive/recurrent thoughts, images or perceptions of the event
- Recurrent distressing dreams of the event
- Acting or feeling as if the event was recurring ("flashbacks")
- Intense psychological distress to cues that symbolize the event, i.e., smells, sounds
- Physiological reactions to symbolic cues

Persistent avoidance of stimuli associated with trauma and numbing of general reactions by three or more:
- Avoid thoughts, feelings, or conversations of event
- Avoid activities/places/people around the event
- Inability to recall important aspects of the trauma
- Marked loss of interest in activities
- Feeling detached from others
- Restricted range of emotion
- Sense of poor future

Symptoms of increased arousal (two or more):
- Difficulty falling/staying asleep
- Irritability/anger
- Difficulty concentrating
- Hypervigilance
- Exaggerated startle response

Chart 6.4

---

many treatment plans continue to bury the scars under layers of compliance programming.

What is PTSD? Perhaps you can recall a traumatic loss that happened five or ten years ago such as loss of job, loss of a loved one, or breakup of a friendship. Today you can remember the unpleasantness, but frankly you now realize that life went on. You have met new people; have a different job, etc. You may even realize that you can't quite remember what all the fuss was about. In posttraumatic stress disorder, however, the individual experiences events that are above and beyond the ordinary. These events would be traumatic to ANYONE (i.e., IQ status is not a disclaimer!). The person remains severely traumatized even years later and the intensity of the feelings does not diminish over time. Their response is one of fear, helplessness, or horror. In children (and possibly non-verbal adults) this may be displayed as disorganized or agitated behavior.

For some people, the event was so traumatic that they couldn't deal with it at the time so the memories are buried. When something happens that begins to retrigger the memories, the walls that hold the memories back come crashing down. Once the walls crash, there is often no putting them back up. People may have flashbacks or nightmares about the trauma. Trigger events might be seeing a child at the same age they were at the time of the abusive situation. The person might hear about similar situations. While both good and negative memories can be triggered through all our senses, the sense of smell is the most powerful memory trigger. People may smell a perfume or cologne worn by their abuser that will trigger the memories. The person may act as if the event were reoccurring. The person will show extreme signs of anxiety. There may even be a numbing of all emotions, sleep disturbance, increased startle response, and hypervigilance (like Al).

Alice is a lady with severe mental retardation who slugged anyone who coughed. As she was essentially nonverbal, people could not figure out what was wrong. Trust me, absenteeism by staff skyrocketed during the cold and flu season. After repeated failed behavior plans, the social worker went digging through the files. It was noted that Alice's father had died of emphysema. When the social worker spoke with Alice's sister, the family secret came tumbling out. Alice's father had beaten Alice regularly. The exertion often caused him to start coughing. The sound of coughing was Alice's trigger. Since that time, Alice has been somewhat desensitized to the sound of coughing, but when she is not feeling well, or is stressed about other issues, I suggest you take your upper respiratory infection elsewhere.

Dr. Ruth Ryan (1993) recommends a six-point protocol for treatment of PTSD. It is presumed that this protocol would also be useful for those persons who have a history of abuse, but without diagnosable PTSD. The protocol includes:

1. Careful use of appropriate medications, but not just medications alone.

2. A complete medical evaluation and treatment of any additional health concerns.

3. Reduce complications of other medications or treatments (i.e., side effects from other medications, in-

sisting the person eat food forced on them by the abuser, etc.).

4. Individual and/or group therapy.

5. Change situations in the environment to avoid triggering events, i.e., stop coughing. A person who is sent to their room as punishment may trigger memories of being locked up in isolation.

6. Lots of staff and family training and support. Front line staffs are unfortunately some of the last ones to learn about PTSD and the first ones to be assaulted when they inadvertently trigger a memory. In addition, I have worked with staff with their own abuse histories, which requires even more caution.

Please note that unless the entire protocol is put into action, successful treatment will probably not happen. A person cannot simply be medicated and expected to improve. I have also witnessed cases where the individual is given "therapy" and then sent back to the abusive situation. Obviously this person got worse instead of better. We become part of the abusing system when we knowingly or unknowingly send a person back to an abuser. The abused person learns to trust no one.

Although I didn't want to add this, I will. All people will recognize abuse, regardless of someone else's determination of their IQ or ability. I add this because I was describing symptoms of PTSD found in a woman said to be profoundly retarded. The person I was talking with stopped me and asked, "How would someone like that even know they had been abused?" This is a misconception that assumes that simply because a person scores low on an intelligence test, she has no feelings, no memories, or more accurately no heart and no mind. Besides believing that some people with disabilities cannot feel, there is the misconception that no one would find "someone like that" physically attractive. Therefore they would never be sexually loved, so if they are violated "someone like that" would not know.

Rape and abuse are about power, control, and violence, not sex. Abusive people most typically prefer victims that have trouble communicating or at least that other people will not believe. Thus the high degree of abuse in persons with developmental disabilities is not because the person has a developmental disability, but simply because there are people who like to abuse and these are ready targets.

I was asked to provide therapy for a young woman with Down syndrome who had been sexually abused for years by a neighbor. The neighbor was not prosecuted and sent to prison when my client's abuse was discovered. He did not go to prison until he had abused "a normal person". This is outrageous for two reasons. First, my client was not believed and not allowed the opportunity to press charges in court because of her disability. Secondly, the other young woman would never have been abused if the abuser had been tried and convicted the first time!

Barbara was 72 years old when we first met. A review of the files indicated that most of her major decompensations happened during July. Nothing useful was in the file to indicate what had happened, so I did the stupid thing and asked Barbara. She promptly screamed that July was a terrible month and ran out of the room.

In spite of staff's best effort, come July, she had a major decompensation and had to be rehospitalized. While there, she began talking about the baby. Since she was also diagnosed with schizophrenia, it was assumed that all of her talk about "the baby" was delusional. Coincidentally there was a staff person there who had known Barbara many years prior. This staff person remembered a story about Barbara having been raped and impregnated. According to Barbara (later told when she was more coherent), when the baby was born, she was told that the baby was dead and she never got to hold it. The baby's birthday was in July. She had never forgotten. Because she was slow and psychotic, all of her talk of babies in danger was disregarded as delusional. (It is important to recall that even when a person is delusional because of a psychotic disorder, he may still have accurate information to offer.)

Following that hospitalization, in the fall of that year, staff gathered to plant bulbs in a garden outside in memory of the baby. Although Barbara gave permission to go on with the planting, she was unable to handle the situation and refused to attend. When spring came, the flowers came up. July came and went that year and she was doing better. At the time of the first book when this story came out, Barbara had continued to do well for some time. She has since been rehospitalized several times because the situation of the abuse and loss of the child continues to compound her other disorders such that full recompensation of her symptoms has never occurred.

Besides the SSRI's (Charts 4.5b & 6.5a) discussed earlier, there are many other anti-anxiety medications on the market. Medications called beta-blockers (6.5b) are usually used to treat high blood pressure. These medications include propranalol (Inderal), nadolol (Corgard), and metaprolol (Lopressor). Beta-blockers work particularly well in the performance anxiety disorders such as fear of speaking in public places and public events. They appear to work by blocking the body's response to the stress hormones in the blood stream. The beta-blockers have also been used for the treatment of rage behaviors and occasionally in treatment resistant bipolar disorder.

It is strongly recommended to have the person evaluated by his primary care physician before initiating beta-blockers. As one would guess, since these medications are primarily prescribed for hypertension, they can have significant effects on the circulatory system. If somebody has anxiety, but doesn't have high blood pressure, we can potentially dangerously lower his or her blood pressure. Persons receiving these medications should have their pulse and blood pressure monitored regularly (no less than weekly). The drug should be held if the pulse rate goes below 60 beats per minute, or if the blood pressure goes below 90/60. Another concern is that a potential side effect of the beta-blockers is depression. Other side effects include dizziness (especially if the person stands too fast), cold hands and feet and occasionally confusion. If the cold hands and feet are severe, or if the person appears confused, contact your doctor immediately. Do not act on your own. These medications should not be stopped suddenly unless directed by your doctor.

The benzodiazepines (Chart 6.5c) as a group have been used for anxiety disorders and occasionally seizure disorders for many, many years. Some people are concerned these medications can cause physical addictions. While that is true, few of the folks I work with are in a position to find illegal sources of medications to fuel an addiction. A physical addiction in this case simply means that the medications should not be stopped abruptly. The gradual weaning process will take time but not nearly as long as it does for some of the older antipsychotic medications. To avoid physical addiction in anyone, recommendations are that these medications should be used only on a short-term basis, but the general community has used them as a long-term response to stress.

Chart 6.5a

Selective serotonin reuptake inhibitors and Effexor have either FDA indications for various anxiety disorders OR are clinically presumed to treat with anxiety disorders.

(See Chart 4.5b for: Celexa, Prozac, Lexapro, Luvox, Paxil, Zoloft.

[1] May take longer to work than when used for depression. May require higher dosages than traditionally used for depression.

When my family was going through a particularly stress-ful time and I found myself dealing with severe stomach pains. I felt so pressed for time, that I wanted a quick "drive-through" form of help. When 3 prescription medi-cations weren't helping my stomach, I had to stop and take a good look at myself. With the help of prayer, friends, relaxation techniques, and finally recognizing the true value of exercise (Boy, I hate that the experts were right!), I was able to stop all the medications. When my stomach starts hurting again, I can generally find that I've stopped doing one or more of the above items. Had I not taken control of my stomach, serious damage could have resulted. One concern with the older anxiety medi-cines is that they work…and work fast. People may not listen to their bodies asking them to slow down.

Most of the benzodiazepines can cause drowsiness. Per-sons taking these medications may have trouble concen-trating, especially initially. This is also a concern for the elderly where the confusion may appear as dementia when in fact it is simply a side effect of the medication. The biggest concern for the benzodiazepines as a group, however, in persons with disabilities is their tendency to disinhibit some people.

Disinhibition means a person acts in a way not usual for them (ie swearing from the pastor's wife), or unaccept-able by others – yelling in the grocery store. If I stand up in front of a large crowd at a presentation and suddenly start to scratch myself in private areas, other people watching may become acutely embarrassed by my activities. It is not socially acceptable for me to comment that a coworker's outfit happens to be the most ugly outfit that I have seen in a long time. I am also not allowed to charge across the mall parking lot and start slugging somebody in the head simply because I don't like the way he parked his car. We all may have these urges to act in socially unacceptable ways at times, but we don't usually act on them. The most common chemical that disinhibits people is the well-known alcohol. We have all heard of calm, gentle, sober people who become mean drunks in the presence of alcohol. The benzodiazepines as a group have a tendency to cause disinhibition particularly when somebody has a known structural defect of the brain such as a closed head injury, history of encephalitis, or many of the other causative agents of mental retardation.

Anxiety Medication Benzodiazepines (usually given in divided dosages)			
Short Acting:			Other uses
alprazolam	Xanax	0.5 - 4 mg/day	panic disorder
lorazepam	Ativan	0.5 - 6 mg/day	seizure control
Long Acting:			
chlordiazepoxide	Librium	5 - 100 mg/day	alcohol detox
clonazepam	Klonopin	0.25 - 2 mg/day	panic disorder, mania, seizure control
diazepam	Valium	2 - 20 mg/day	seizure control

Common side effects - all can cause disinhibition, drowsiness, impaired coordination, and cognitive difficulties.

Chart 6.5c

As discussed in an earlier chapter, the frontal lobe is traditionally considered to be the portion of the brain (located just behind your forehead) that is responsible for attention and impulse control. When somebody has diminished frontal lobe functioning from a closed head injury, ADHD, or other neurological insults, he or she is far more likely to be disinhibited with or without medication. While the benzodiazepams are strongly recommended in treatment of acute agitation/aggression, their long-term usage in persons with a disability may create disinhibited aggression...not a pretty sight!

Sometimes people have been given short acting anti-anxiety medications (that is, they work within minutes and last only a few hours) to help them with medical procedures. I sometimes wonder, however, if we aren't further traumatizing people by reducing their ability to fight frightening situations. Let's face it, if you have been sexually abused, a gynecological appointment is not a fun time. We should not wonder then when a person who is nonverbal screams, and races out of the room when the doctor attempts to get a Pap smear. Some innovative programs now recognize these issues and will take as many appointments as necessary to help a person with her fears before doing the Pap smear. When such programs are not available or an option, consideration should be given to what is more important . . . the fright of the test or the potential risk of not doing the test. Since there is no universal answer for this, each situation must be considered on its merits.

I had the misfortune of seeing Helen in a very black and blue state. She looked like she had been run over by a dump truck, but Helen had done all of the damage herself. At age 60, she was long past the time of having monthly menstrual cycles. When she began experiencing some uterine bleeding, a Pap smear was warranted. The doctor was female, very gentle, and took quite a lot of time assisting Helen during the Pap smear. That night, however, in the quiet of her room, Helen beat herself mercilessly until staff happened to make a go-around and saw the blood on the sheets. Further investigation into the history noted that this lady had a history of abuse prior to the institutional setting and that possibly continued while in the institutional setting. Her response to the Pap smear was seen as traumatic and tragic, but unfortunately not unusual.

Another concern with the short acting benzodiazepines is when an individual has an anxiety disorder and feels anxious all the time. A short acting anxiety medicine helps a person feel better for two to four hours at a time and then the medication washes out. They are then given another dose of the medication (something such as Ativan is typically given two to three times a day) and they feel better for several hours and again it washes out of their system. It is as if they are on the anxiety merry-go-round that never seems to take a stop. In these instances, a better option may be a longer acting benzodiazepine such as clonazepam.

Generally, however, even though they initially take longer to provide relief, the drugs of choice for most anxiety disorders are the SSRI's used for depression. When SSRI's were first used in persons with depression, it was noted that they felt less depressed AND less anxious. A new era of treatment began. Unfortunately as stated in Chapter 4, the SSRI's and another anti-anxiety medication very similar to the antidepressants, buspirone (BuSpar) takes several weeks at therapeutic dosages to reach their optimal effect. As a matter of fact in the case of OCD, we do not say that an SSRI is ineffective until at least three months at the same dosage has gone by. The person may only need 20 mg of Prozac but it may take a full 90 days before the desired effect starts to be obtained. Some consideration has also been given to gabapentin (Neurontin), and very low dosages of the newer atypical antipsychotics.

As with Depression, people with anxiety disorders get locked into harmful thought patterns. Unless these thought patterns are challenged in a therapeutic setting, the medications are often only partially effective. Individual and group therapy often provide as much relief, if not more, than medications. Unfortunately, many health plans do not pay for the therapy. In addition, when advocating for persons with disabilities, many support people, therapists, and even systems fail to recognize the importance of developing more effective coping strategies such as relaxation techniques. In this regard, the field of disabilities has been lacking. We have not looked at enough research-based therapy programs to address the questions of the money counters. Most of us providing therapy can point out many successes, but research is still required.

Other Anxiety Medications

| clomipramine (Used for OCD) | Anafranil | 25 - 250 mg/day |

Common side effects - drowsiness, constipation, dry mouth, tremor, dizziness, sweating, GI upset, weight gain, and sexual dysfunction.

| buspirone | Buspar | 10 - 60 mg/day |

Common side effects - mild sedation, GI upset, headache, dizziness.

| beta - blockers | propranolol | Inderal |
| | nadolol | Corgard |

Chart 6.5b

Chapter 7

Schizophrenia

Psalms 13:2a:
How long must I wrestle with my thoughts and
everyday have sorrow in my heart?

Charles was one of the most distinguished persons that I have ever known. He was only 22 when we met, yet he had that kind of quiet confidence that you sense when you are with someone who knows his own worth. He didn't talk much, and that's what really bothered people. He was referred to me because people thought he was psychotic.

Charles has Down syndrome. He lived in a group home that had been classified "behavioral." I met Charles in 1984 before the nature of psychiatric illness in persons with developmental disabilities was well understood. Even so, I never quite understood why he was in that particular home. All of the other people in his home were aggressive, self-destructive, or loud. His very silence made him stand out.

Although Charles wasn't aggressive, he would occasionally put on a fifty-cent plastic sheriff's badge, and scribble in a notebook. After writing, he would say "humph!" then neatly put his things away. Surely, staff reasoned, this was weird, delusional, behavior.

Schizophrenia is the granddaddy of all psychiatric disorders. As the Psalm above implies, it involves irrational thoughts, mood problems, and often a dismantling of the core person. Historically, more people with disabilities have been labeled "schizophrenic" than any other diagnosis. Or, when people wanted to be a bit more vague and perhaps more accurate, they would use the term "psychotic disorder, NOS" (Not Otherwise Specified). The ability to diagnose these real illnesses in persons with disabilities remains extremely difficult, if not often impossible. Although the antipsychotic medications continue to be the most commonly prescribed class of drugs for persons with developmental disabilities, schizophrenia is probably the least frequently observed disorder in this group.

What is schizophrenia? Some of you have seen the bumper sticker that reads, "You are never alone when you are schizophrenic". Although I am sure great thought goes into bumper sticker writing, "schizo", or the split, is actually a split from reality, not split personality or multiple personality disorder. Persons with schizophrenia lose the ability to recognize real life from the often-frightening drama going on inside their heads. Imagine if you will, Mark.

"I'm locked up in my room, but people can still watch me. I can see eyes coming through the heat vents. I tried closing the curtains, but the radio waves continue to zoom at me from Mars. There is no safe place. I hear the pounding at the door. My father, or somebody, who looks like my father — I can never be quite certain who it might be, is insisting I come out and eat dinner. Food? Who can think of food at a time like this? Everyone's out to get me. The dangers are out there untold. I can hear all these people talking. Where are they coming from? Why can't I see them? Nobody else seems to see them yet I hear them all the time especially when I try to sleep. There is no need to shave or bathe. There is no need for anything since the radio waves continue to control my every action. Why don't they understand? Why don't I understand?"

While "Mark's" thoughts are actually a summary of thoughts relayed to me by many people, they could easily be the thoughts of any individual with schizophrenia. These frightening symptoms of hearing voices and believing bizarre things often prompt initial referrals for treatment.

When resent studies looked at the early developmental years of persons with schizophrenia after the diagnosis has been made, they saw some similar patterns. The signs are often so vague, however, as to be unnoticeable, or at least not readily attributed to forthcoming problems. Other people with schizophrenia often appeared "okay" in childhood. In either event, the disease typically strikes people in the prime of their youth. "Unignorable" symptoms begin for most people in their late teens to early 20's, which devastate individual lives and families.

Gradually as the illness takes over, the person becomes more isolative. He may become frightened of even familiar people. She no longer performs self-care, almost as if she no longer recognizes the need for self-care. He may hear voices that seem more real than the people that are actually there. She may begin to firmly believe very bizarre things. The symptoms of schizophrenia (chart 7.1) are generally divided into the positive symptoms such as delusions, hallucinations, and odd speech; and negative symptoms: flat affect, lack of enjoyment, poor eye contact, and inability to begin or stay with activities.

We all gain information of our worlds through our senses. Sometimes our senses play tricks on us that are called illusions. An illusion is a misperception of a real stimulus. For example, on a hot day, the pavement ahead of your car may look wet. No matter how fast you drive up to the 'wet spot'; it magically dries up by the time you get there. Or, if you have ever been alone in a house on a rainy night, you might think that the wind in the trees was a burglar trying to break in. This is not a psychotic, abnormal understanding of the outside world. In each

> ## *Characteristic Symptoms of Schizophrenia , (DSM IV-TR)*
>
> A. Two or more of the following:
>   - Delusions.
>   - Hallucinations.
>   - Disorganized speech.
>   - Very disorganized behavior or total lack of movement (catatonia).
>   - Negative symptoms (flat or inappropriate affect, lack of pleasure, poor eye contact, inability to initiate or persist in activities.
>
> B. Social or occupational dysfunction or very diminished self-care.

Chart 7.1

of these examples, other people could receive the same information through their senses (sight, hearing, taste, touch, or smell) and understand your misinterpretations. Indeed magicians would be out of a job if not for illusionary work.

Persons suffering from schizophrenia, however, are unable to trust their five senses. They may hear, see, taste, smell or feel things that are not based in the real world. These are hallucinations. Hearing voices that no one else hears is the most common, but hallucinations can involve any of the senses. Occasionally, the voices are friendly, but most often the voices are very frightening. Imagine being unable to determine if what you are hearing is coming from the outside world or coming from your own internal world. Who do you believe? Generally it is the loudest voice. Unfortunately for persons with schizophrenia, the loudest voice typically is the internal one.

Like "Mark", people suffering from schizophrenia often experience bizarre beliefs called delusions. A delusion, by definition, is a false fixed belief that no amount of logic can change. These beliefs may include that the television or radio has special messages just for them. They may believe that the secret police are following them. They may believe that they have special magical powers. Often the delusions are of a paranoid nature: they believe that others are out to get them. The delusions and hallucinations can blend together to form a very intricate network of fears and irrational behaviors.

If I firmly believe that my next-door neighbor is actually a foreign spy who is trying to kill me, I am highly unlikely to invite her over for a can of diet Pepsi. Now suppose that the next-door neighbor who is unsuspecting of my fears comes over to borrow the garden hose. I might run from her, or even attack in self-defense. Suppose I live in a group home with staff. When staffs try to convince me that the neighbor is simply a nice lady needing to borrow a garden hose, I would certainly begin to mistrust them as well. Thus the circle of mistrust grows until it includes almost everyone I meet.

Whenever I work with people who are currently psychotic (that is experiencing delusions and/or hallucinations for whatever reasons- schizophrenia is not the only cause!), I always try to find out the nature of their delusions and/ or hallucinations. I want to find out if they are a danger to themselves or others. For example, I need to find out if the voices are telling them to harm themselves or to harm someone else. The rate of suicide is very high among persons with schizophrenia, even more so than persons with depression, as it is tragically common for the voices to tell them to hurt themselves.

Once I find out whether they are a danger to themselves or others, I neither agree with their delusions (or hallucinations) nor do I argue with them. By definition, a delusion is not swayed by others' logic. By agreeing with them, I deny their attempts to grasp reality. By arguing with them, I further their distrust in the world and me. Typically, if a person appears frightened, I acknowledge his fear and try to help him feel safe. Remember that emotions are valid no matter their source.

The positive symptoms of schizophrenia have a tendency to increase and decrease during the lifespan of the illness. For example, during serious points in this illness, or the sicker a person becomes, the stranger his conversations. The person who is acutely ill with schizophrenia looses the ability to use abstract thinking and resorts to a more concrete form of thought processing. The standard test to determine the ability to think abstractly is to ask a person to explain a proverb such as "people in glass houses shouldn't throw stones". An abstract answer to this proverb is "don't accuse others of what you are doing." While there could be many other philosophical answers to this proverb, the person thinking concretely will answer, "You shouldn't throw stones because windows will break".

When I worked in a psychiatric hospital, my initial assessment question was always "what brought you here?" If the person began to explain about the problems they were having, I knew that that person could think at least somewhat abstractly. A person with acute schizophrenia, however, would answer concretely "the bus", or "a car". This allowed me to proceed with my assessment accordingly.

Using proverbs or searching for other signs of abstract thinking may be a difficult if not impossible test for persons with intellectual challenges. In non-intellectually challenged children, abstract reasoning begins around the ages of 12 – 14. Younger children will always answer concretely. The "Amelia Bedilia" stories become humorous for older children as they recognize her concrete thinking. When Amelia is asked to dust the living room, she gets out dusting powder and sprays it all around. She mutters, "that's strange, most people would *undust* the furniture!" For individuals with intellectual disabilities, they may never reach that scholastic/maturational age of 12 - 14. Therefore, they will always respond to the proverb interpretation with a concrete answer. Here I would have to know their ability to abstract and then test against their ability rather than frustrate by testing their disability.

Other changes in conversation with a person with schizophrenia will include tangential speech. The person may string many sentences, words or even sounds together that appear totally unrelated. The person may even make up their own words that have meaning only to them. The person may refuse to speak at all. In general, the less amount of time that a person can talk on one concrete subject, such as what they had for breakfast, the sicker they are.

Again, when reading this, remember that people with disabilities may sound as if they have similar problems with speech, but their difficulties are likely related to the disability, not to a psychiatric disorder. It is important to know what their previous level of speaking abilities was and then measure it against what they are currently doing. Thus the importance of family, friends, and staff that know the individual is paramount when reporting the discrepancies in the current presentation as opposed to the long-standing nature of the disability.

The negative symptoms of schizophrenia include flat (absent) or inappropriate affect (facial expression), lack of pleasure in activities (anhedonia), poor eye contact, an inability to initiate or persist in activities, as well as diminished social or occupational functioning, and cognitive difficulties. In schizophrenia, the person's facial expressions, or lack of them can be very frightening to those around him. The person is often described as having a flat or blunted affect. This means that little emotional content is showing in their nonverbal facial expression. When we interact with others, we generally gain feedback from the other person by facial and body expressions. The person with schizophrenia has very little ability to react to or express abstract feeling states. Although the person may laugh or cry, often inappropriately (such as laugh when told the their favorite relative died), their face shows little or no emotion.

Even when the voices are gone, persons with schizophrenia have extreme difficulty beginning or maintaining activities apparently unrelated to effects of the older antipsychotic medications. This may present as difficulty attending a therapy group or looking for gainful employment. With encouragement, the person might get to work, but unless supported in that arena, the individual may have trouble maintaining the efforts. This is not laziness or poor upbringing; it is a function of the cognitive/executive functioning difficulties caused by the disease. Executive functioning is the dimension of our brain that allows us to organize our day. Upon wakening, I can realize it is Tuesday, I need to go to work, and the children must go to school. In the next 90 minutes typical chaos reigns, but we are all out the door dressed, fed, and with the right supplies. Imagine the chaos if this planning ability is gone.

I recall a story where a medical doctor had had a stroke that resulted in death of a portion of the brain that controlled executive functioning. Tragically, following the stroke, the doctor woke up one night and realized he had a headache. Rather than go to the medicine cabinet in his bathroom, he walked across the street to the hospital where he used to work. A midnight nurse found him helping himself to the hospital supply of aspirin wearing nothing but his lower pajamas and socks. For this doctor, the stroke caused the problems. In schizophrenia, there is a chronic dismantling of the executive functioning aspects of the brain. I recently adjusted the medications of a man who had been working on his Ph.D. in physics when illness struck. He now has trouble organizing his day to fit in getting dressed, making meals, and attending group twice a week.

If one looks at the DSM IV-TR, one will note that there are several different subtypes of schizophrenia where one or more of the above positive or negative symptoms are seen more prominently. The course, severity and duration of any of these subtypes can vary with the individual. Some people have a single episode of schizophrenia that either spontaneously goes away (rarely), or is successfully treated with medications. More people have periodic episodes of this illness throughout their lives that require treatment. They may have residual difficulties in between acute flare-ups, but overall they are able to function to some degree. Unfortunately, many people with schizophrenia, even with current treatment options, are never able to return to their pre-illness level of functioning. In these cases, it is often the negative symptoms that impair the individual the most.

There are many theories surrounding the cause(s) of schizophrenia. Historical beliefs have included everything from Satan invading the individual or their parents to improper toilet training. Current research suggests that the brain of an individual with schizophrenia had structural abnormalities even before the onset of symptoms. For example, there are certain fluid-filled spaces within all brains. In people with schizophrenia, these spaces are larger, giving rise to the idea that even before symptoms start, brain tissue has already been altered. Another theory suggests that the connections between brain cells set up chaotic pathways. It may be that the different structure was a result of embryonic insult such as a viral infection in the mother during critical times of the pregnancy, altered genetics (risk of schizophrenia increases from 1:100 to 1:10 if a close relative has schizophrenia), or other unknown causes. As we discussed in earlier chapters of the book, when the structure is altered, the chemical transport system is altered. Currently, much money, research, and time are being spent in studying the structural/functional aspects of the brain along with the chemical neurotransmission disorders in schizophrenia.

Prior to World War II, once a person was diagnosed with schizophrenia, little was known to help, and people were generally locked up in institutional settings for life. Lobotomies (removal of part of the brain), insulin shock therapy (inducing brief coma from low blood sugar), ice water baths and other "therapies" were tried. While they seem barbaric in today's world, they were signs of desperate practitioners trying to help others in desperate positions. (Fortunately, these therapies have since been abandoned.)

The first medications to arrive in psychiatry were referred to as major tranquilizers (compared to Valium that was labeled a minor tranquilizer). In the 1950's when major tranquilizers were first realized to have use in psychiatry, it was believed that people were psychotic because of their difficulties dealing with fear and anxiety surrounding their upbringing. It was hoped that if we could simply unravel the person down far enough to find the core of their dysfunction, we would be able to provide the correct one-on-one personal therapy that would then cure the disorder. In the meantime, the medications were used to "calm" the individual down.

The discovery that medications could even help came about quite by accident. Prior to the days of human rights committees, when an individual with schizophrenia was placed in an institution, they basically lost all rights as a human being. Many, many drug trials were conducted in facilities for persons with disabilities as well as persons with mental illness. A medication by the name of chlorpromazine came under investigation. Persons in mental institutions were put through all kinds of drug studies. Chlorpromazine proved to be relatively ineffective for what they were looking for. Some astute staff at the institutions, however, began to notice that some of these drug trial participants no longer appeared as psychotic. They seemed able to function better. These individuals often "calmed down;" hence came the name "major tranquilizer." Chlorpromazine, or Thorazine as it is better known, became widely prescribed in psychiatry throughout the world. Thioridazine (Mellaril) followed closely behind as well as many other classical antipsychotic medications. (Chart 7.2)

As study into schizophrenia continued, scientists considered that if a biochemical agent such as chlorpromazine was able to create a functional difference in an individual, perhaps there was a biochemical disorder within the body in the first place. Perhaps, it was reasoned, schizophrenia had nothing to do with toilet training at all. Because Thorazine, Mellaril, and Haldol were known in laboratory settings to be strong blockers of dopamine, and they had the effects of decreasing delusions and hallucinations, initial research looked no further. In addition, the higher dosages could stop almost any aggressive behavior. It was never imagined, however, that these individuals could become productive members of their worlds again.

Unlike the serotonin theories in depression where the brain cell was deficient in serotonin, schizophrenia was believed to be caused by an excess of dopamine flooding the next cell. That is, if nerve cell #1 (refer back to the nerve cell drawing in Chapter 4) required 100 dopamines to transmit a signal from nerve cell #1 to nerve cell #2, people with schizophrenia, were hypothetically sending across 150 or even 200 little dopamine transmitters. This excess then built up in the space between the nerve cells allowing for nerve cells to fire off of their own accord without any external stimulus from the outside.

Older Antipsychotic/Neuroleptic (D₂ Blocker) Medications Chart 7.2			
	DOSAGE RANGE	EPS [1]	ANTI-C [2]
LOW POTENCY			
chlorpromazine (Thorazine)	300 - 800 mg/day	X	XXX
thioridazine (Mellaril)	100 - 600 mg/day	X	XXX
loxapine [3] (Loxitane)	10 - 250 mg/day	XX	XX
perphenazine (Trilafon)	4 - 40 mg/day	XX	XX
mesoridazine (Serentil)	25 - 200 mg/cay	XX	XX
HIGH POTENCY			
fluphenazine (Prolixin)	1 - 20 mg/day	XXX	X
haloperidol (Haldol)	1 - 20 mg/day	XXX	X
thiothixene (Navane)	4 - 60 mg/day	XXX	X
trifluoperazine (Stelazine)	2 - 20 mg/day	XXX	X

[1] Extrapyramidal Side Effects: akathesia, Parkinsonism, and/or dystonia

[2] Anticholinergic Side Effects: Drowsiness, constipation, blurry vision, delayed urnination, sexual dysfunctions, and/or dry mouth.

[3] Considered by some to have "atypical" properties

The older antipsychotics such as Haldol, Mellaril, Thorazine, etc., work by plugging up the receptor sites in the next nerve cell. This way even though the first nerve cell continues to pound out presumed extra dopamine; it is less likely to initiate signals in the second nerve cell.

Virtually all antipsychotics with D2 (dopamine 2) blockade properties are equally as effective in stopping the positive symptoms of schizophrenia – the delusions, hallucinations, garbled speech, etc. (Equally effective in large research groups, but individuals will respond differently to specific drugs!) Unfortunately, there are several problems with this more simple theory and practice of dopamine blockade.

My husband works on all our cars. Our 1989 car required 3 different starters over our many driving years together. Although it should have been easy to replace (at least he SAID it should be easy), the starter was located just out of easy reach such that it was almost impossible to fix. I remember bandaging many ripped fingers, covering the girls' ears (from the assistive language), and running to the parts stores for extra whatzits during the repairs. What seems simple to replace in theory is often difficult in reality.

First of all, like the changing of a simple car part, the specific part of the brain that needs assistance isn't always easy to get to. Medications that impact on the brain must cross what's called the blood-brain barrier. I may never understand why alcohol and street drugs can cross immediately, but potentially helpful medicines take so much longer. In addition, as any car mechanic can tell you, the minute you start to move some parts around, you may mess up other parts of the car. D2 receptors are found in at least 4 different pathways of the brain, and the older antipsychotics are very unconcerned with which ones they block, thus resulting in many undesired side effects. The second time the starter was replaced in our car, we discovered that the transmission was going bad and had to be replaced too. In this case, repair of one section of the car uncovered other more extensive problems. Likewise, although the symptoms of delusions and hallucinations often responded well to these older medications, the negative symptoms of schizophrenia such as inability to initiate or maintain occupational activities rarely did. Indeed these symptoms worsened, but worsening was accepted as the price tag associated with the treatment.

As time went on, clinicians realized that the negative symptoms of schizophrenia although not as flamboyant as believing staff were space aliens, were actually the predictors of worse outcome. In my favorite movie of all time, (Miracle on 34th Street) Kris Kringle is considered 'crazy' because he believes he is Kris Kringle, AKA, Santa Claus. In other areas of his life, however, he is quite functional. Indeed, he finds an ideal job, a place to stay, and develops sincere friendships. He is placed in a hospital only when he is agitated because others don't believe him. I won't ruin the ending for those 3 people out there who have never seen it, but unusual beliefs do not predict outcome. For persons beyond the walls of Hollywood with truly false fixed beliefs, many continue to function within their worlds.

Apart from their use in treating schizophrenia, in the 1950's, the older antipsychotic medications made their entry into facilities for persons with developmental disabilities. As the 60's rolled into the 70's and 80's, we began to recognize that we could not simply chemically straitjacket people with disabilities who displayed normal reactions (AKA: aggression) to the abnormality of life in an institution. Indeed the twisted paradox of bureaucracies meant that medication was used NOT for the people with true psychiatric illness, but often for those without! Since people with disabilities were not allowed to be mentally ill at this time, and the negative side effects of the medicines were becoming more noticeable, systems all over tried to abolish these medicines for persons with disabilities overnight. The resulting tardive withdrawal syndrome discussed later in this chapter made people rethink these ideas.

To justify the continued use of these medicines in persons with aggression, we tried to find behaviors that looked like symptoms of schizophrenia. We noted that these individuals talked to themselves. They were aggressive. They may have yelled uncontrollably. They were aggressive. They used concrete thinking. They were aggressive. Sometimes their self-care was terrible. They were aggressive. They might not sleep well. They were aggressive. With all these things going on, well, they must have schizophrenia or Psychotic Disorder NOS. And thus, these diagnoses (once we conceded that psychiatry had a place in disabilities) became the number one psychiatric misdiagnosis for people with intellectual challenges.

Jack frustrated the people he lived and worked with. Jack used to be able to navigate the bus system well. He even taught others in his home how to ride the bus system. When he wouldn't leave his room, he lost his job. Jack was almost ready for his own apartment, but now he tells staff that "a man in a white car" keeps following him. His job used to allow him to buy a very fashionable wardrobe. The day we met, he had on ripped shorts, two sweaters and mismatched boots. He had refused to change saying, "President Nixon wants me to wear these." Staff complained that Jack continually told stories. Even if staff caught him repeatedly in his lies, Jack continued to tell them as if they were true.

Although Jack does have schizophrenia along with mild mental retardation, many attributes of a person with disabilities (minus the aggression which is NOT a direct attribute of having a disability, but rather a tragically common reaction to uncommon stressors) such as concrete thinking have been misconstrued as symptoms of schizophrenia. People may report to the psychiatrist that the person with developmental disabilities talks to himself. No one else can see whom that person is talking to. Well, this may or may not be a problem and it may or may not be psychotic.

If you have children, have you ever heard yourself coming out of their mouths? We live in the country. Many years ago I was making supper when my then 2-year old insisted, "Go outside? Go outside?!" I told her no. I didn't want her wandering out in the backfield by herself. A little while later, I heard her on the stairs talking. She held two dolls, one in each hand. Doll #1asked repeatedly; "Go outside? Go outside?" Doll #2 screamed, "No. No." I obviously sounded a lot meaner to her than I had intended. By refusing to let her go out, I created a situation that she found stressful. While role-playing with her dolls, she was able to work out some of her angered feelings independently.

"We" say people with developmental disabilities are developmentally delayed. In its simplest form, this means that the person may still use coping strategies found at earlier levels of development. Again, I am not implying that these are somehow children in adult bodies, but rather they may not have learned advanced coping strategies given their situations. Please recall that the rest of us don't necessarily use adult-like coping strategies either. (Such as resisting the 55 MPH speed limitation by driving 59 MPH) When an individual with a developmental disability is talking to himself, he may be reenacting a stressful situation and dealing with the feelings much as my daughter did on the day she wanted to go outside.

A person living in a group home situation, who is bored or feels left out, might talk to a friend that no one else sees. This is not psychotic behavior. These behaviors may, in fact, be very useful for the individual. As the person grows, develops and gains real friends, and also learns new improved ways to cope, these behaviors may disappear. Maybe not, I still talk to myself when I am busy working on a project. I figure I am one of the few people that I know of that actually listens to me.

Another complicating factor when attempting to diagnose schizophrenia in a person with intellectual disabilities is observed behaviors that may appear to the outsider as a psychotic behavior. Flashbacks of previous traumatic experiences may very well include visual or auditory hallucinations. Unfortunately, these sights and sounds are very reality based, old reality, but reality nonetheless. The use of antipsychotic medications may in fact delay the healing process.

People wondered if Shelly was psychotic. She often looked very frightened. During these times, she had a blank look on her face and would scream "No, No!" Since several other concerns indicated the possibility of abuse, her past was reviewed. Not only had she been victimized in the institution, she had also been sexually abused by several family members prior to entering the institution. (According to the intake statement, she was originally placed in the institution after her family could no longer handle her "sudden aggressive behavior".) Shelly was experiencing visual and auditory hallucinations of her past. As opposed to a psychotic break, however, her hallucinations could better be understood as very real, very present memories. Treatment required for Shelly was described in the previous chapter.

At this time, if I work with someone with less than a high moderate range of mental retardation who is reported to be hearing voices, I am very, very hesitant to diagnose him with schizophrenia. The person has got to be able to conceptualize to me that the voices that they are hearing are something that are not of this world. The typical conversation that I have had with many people who are thought to be schizophrenic sounds like this: "Do you hear voices?"

"Yes!"

"Whose voices are you hearing?"

"Yours."

"No. No. No. Are you hearing any voices of somebody who is not here in this room?"

"Yes."

"Whose voices are you hearing?"

"The people in the room next door."

When I finally get to, "Is this voice that you are hearing something that nobody else could hear if they were sitting here but is not somebody that is sitting in the other room?" the results become questionable. The questions have necessarily become abstract in order to get information, but then cannot be answered. It then becomes paramount to look for some of the other symptomatology that goes with schizophrenia such as the *regression* of self care, difficulty dealing with other people, flattened affect, and delusional thinking. And just to complicate issues, remember that just because you may not understand or like what a person is saying, does not make the idea delusional. Or simply put, the person may be relaying factual information that others do not want to hear. (Talking about abusive episodes, behavior of staff or other subjects uncomfortable for the listener, but a reality for the speaker).

Jack, unlike Shelly, clearly had schizophrenia. People could identify losses in function. However, indicators are seldom this clear. In general, a diagnosis of schizophrenia in persons with developmental disabilities should be considered as a last choice, not first, for safety's sake. Am I therefore declaring that there should be a total ban on the antipsychotic medications? No. NO. And NO! These medications are extremely important to persons with schizophrenia. We are now recognizing the even greater role of the newer atypical antipsychotic medications (Chart 7.3) for many other disorders. These medications can have far-reaching effects, which is good when one considers how debilitating schizophrenia can be. I simply object to using medications to restrict a person's growth, while at the same time potentially not addressing their real needs, as would happen when one misdiagnoses schizophrenia and overlooks the true diagnosis.

Since aggression either towards self, others or property can be dangerous, and medications seem to control it sometimes, why is using these medications such a big deal? I suspect that if I suggested removing some of the individuals that you are working with from their Haldol or

Mellaril, you might be more inclined to leave a hate letter in my mailbox. Let's be honest. How many of you think that the person in question based on the above criteria is really and truly schizophrenic? What is the fear or the real concern of what would happen if they'd come off of the medication? The person might become (more) aggressive.

Let's look at the reality of what could happen therapeutically or non-therapeutically in the presence of these medications. As indicated before, the older antipsychotic medications as a group are dopamine 2 blockers. The antipsychotics fill in the dopamine 2 receptor spots, so the dopamine cannot activate the next cell. In this way, for the person with schizophrenia, even though the cells either produce too much dopamine or are overly sensitive to dopamine, the next cell is not triggered when it shouldn't be.

When this blockade is put into effect in a person without schizophrenia, the brain cells are really compromised especially for a person with cognitive difficulties. Remember dopamine is involved in the thought pathways of the brain. When a dopamine blockade is put into place, normal signals for thinking, feeling, reasoning, and understanding the world are reduced. It's sort of like telling somebody to sort a laundry basket full of dark socks and then turning out the lights!

Besides decreased cognition, the older antipsychotics as a group are not very specific and can create many side effects even for those persons who do need these medications. The older dopamine blockers cannot distinguish between the dopamine pathways in which they should work from the ones in which they shouldn't. Since Dopamine is found in at least 4 major brain pathways, serious side effects occur when these pathways are blocked. In addition, much like my husband working on our old car, the minute you begin adjusting one part, you start twisting and turning on other parts and suddenly find a part in the back broken loose. When you start adjusting any chemical within the brain, you may also inadvertently start adjusting other chemicals within the brain in either a positive or a negative way.

Tardive Dyskinesia (TD) is an often-irreversible side effect of the older (and possibly newer) antipsychotic medications. TD usually develops after the person has been taking the medication for an extended period of time. Some people, however, develop TD after only a short time on the medication. People most susceptible to the development of Tardive Dyskinesia include the elderly, particularly women past menopause, and those with diabetes.

Esther celebrated her 66th birthday recently. The cake was a little smaller than she would have liked, but her blood sugars for diabetes are hard to keep in range. She'd been on Haldol for many, many, many, many years. Both the psychiatrist and myself had been exceedingly concerned about the use of Haldol in this lady for what seemed to be behavioral control. In addition to the diabetes, Esther is also diagnosed with severe mental retardation, and she is deaf. Because she is over 60 years of age, the concerns regarding Tardive Dyskinesia became more and more prominent.

We attempted to reduce the Haldol, but she became more withdrawn and hit her face to the point of swelling and bruising. No medical cause could be found. We tried an antidepressant suspecting that the tears and the withdrawal had something to do with depression. She became more agitated. The pounding of her face became more severe. She even appeared to be seeing things that no one else could see. This is one of those cases where the minute you say, "always be suspicious that something might not be a psychotic process" it shows up. Unfortunately, the older antipsychotic medication had to be increased, but again the concerns of tardive dyskinesia continued.

It is fortunate for us, and particularly for this lady, that in the last few years, several medications referred to as atypical or novel antipsychotic medications have been released. These medications do continue to provide some dopamine blockade but at a significantly lower level then the older antipsychotic medications. They seem to do it to a sufficient degree, however, to block the presence of delusions and hallucinations experienced by many people with schizophrenia. In addition to this, they act on a variety of other neurotransmitters within the brain. This combined action seems to reduce the dopamine blockade in the movement pathway, thus significantly reducing the

Atypical Antipsychotics
Chart 7.3

Generic	Trade Name	Dosage Range	EPS	Sedation	Antichol	Weight Gain
Aripiprazole	Abilify	10-30 mg/day	+/-	+/-	0	+/-
Clozapine	Clozaril	300-900 mg/day	+/-	++++	++++	+++
Olanzapine	Zyprexa	5-20 mg/day	+	++	++	+++
Risperidone	Risperdal	0.25-6 mg/day	++	+	+	++
Quetiapine	Seroquel	150-750 mg/day	+/-	+++	+	++
Ziprasidone	Geoden	40-160 g/day	+/-	+/-	0	0

Must still montior for EPS/TD, blood glucose changes, EKG changes, neuroleptic malignant syndrome.

risk of tardive dyskinesia. In addition, the multiple actions of these medications have been found to be far more effective in the treatment of the negative symptomatology and even some of the cognitive impairment associated with chronic schizophrenia.

Clozapine (Clozaril) is considered to be the most important breakthrough in the treatment of schizophrenia since Thorazine. It was actually first released in the 70's but quickly pulled from the US market due to potential problems with reducing the body's infection fighters — white blood cells (WBC). As the problems and concerns with schizophrenia continued, it was reintroduced. To avoid potentially life-threatening decline in WBC's, the US Food and Drug Administration (FDA) would only release it in one-week dosages following weekly blood draws. Close monitoring of WBC's is required. (Blood draws can be decreased to every 2 weeks after one year of continuous treatment.) In spite of the cost of the drug, staff time, and lab work, the overwhelming response by sufferers of schizophrenia soon proved that it was a VERY cost-effective form of treatment. People considered hopelessly ill were now able to leave the hospital, rejoin families, even live independently and work! Side effects include serious weight gain, blood pressure changes, drooling and lethargy. In spite of these, most that tried it were very relieved.

As strange as it may seem, not everyone was thrilled. Jeff was hospitalized at age 17. He had always struggled in school, and never returned to finish high school following his first psychotic break. Over the next 3 decades, he spent over 25 of those years in hospital settings. When I first met him, he was receiving over 1400 mg. of Thorazine (usual dosage is 300 – 800 mg/day), and was still very delusional. Approximately 2 years before we met, he had been given IQ testing. At age 47, he was newly diagnosed as "mildly mentally retarded" and moved to a "DD" institution. Whether he was initially intellectually challenged, testing was invalid, or he experienced cognitive decline as a function of severe schizophrenia I do not know. When he was 49, however, he was moved to a community home and started on Clozaril. His illness cleared up with remarkable speed...until he considered suicide. He said later that he "looked in the mirror, and I realized that I'm not 17 anymore. Where did my life go? I can't live like this."

In spite of reactions like Jeff's, most people respond favorably. Given the intensive need for lab work and staff time, other medications that also acted on several transmitters, thus also called "atypical", were soon released. These include Risperidal (risperidone), Zyprexa (olanzapine), Seroquel (quetiapine), and Geodon (ziprasidone). The most recently released medication in the US is Abilify (aripiprazole). This drug works differently from even the "atypicals". It is called a partial-agonist of dopamine. The chemical properties are for the chemists, but in practice it should help with the symptoms of schizophrenia, while actually helping the dopamine process in the movement pathways of the brain.

When Risperidone was initially released, directions for starting it included going from 1 to 6 mg in 3 days and up to a high of 16 mg/day. Many people had unnecessary reactions due to the higher dosages. At higher dosages, it floods out the movement pathway with too much dopamine blockade like the older antipsychotics and may cause the same movement problems seen with the older medications. Current research recommends a much slower dosing schedule, and usually no more than 6 mg/day. At these lower dosages, irregular movements or "EPS" are fairly infrequent. Although weight gain can be seen with this medicine, it is less likely than with some of the other atypicals. It is available in a liquid, and rapid dissolving tablet. Risperidol Consta was recently released by the FDA as the first atypical in a long-term injection format. (Until this point, the only injection format for long-term usage was Haldol and Prolixin Decanoates, both older medications with all the other problems.) Research has shown improved frontal lobe functioning with this medicine. This improved executive functioning has allowed many to resume independent function. On the potentially negative side, Risperidone is associated with increase prolactin levels, which is also a problem with the older antipsychotics. Prolactin is a hormone in the body. Increased prolactin can impair menses in women and increase growth of breast tissue in males along with reduced sexual drive. Whether this has any long-term irreversible effect is unknown. While not currently FDA approved, there are many reports that very low dosages (less than 2 mg.) of Risperidal have a positive effect for some persons with anxiety disorders, depression, and difficulties associated with autism.

Olanzapine (Zyprexa) was the next atypical released. It probably requires a higher dosage (10 – 20 mg/day) than originally thought. Besides schizophrenia, it also has FDA approval for treatment of mania in Bipolar disorder (and initial research suggests it helps with the depressive symptoms in Bipolar disorder as well). Olanzapine has been associated with weight gain. Whether this is entirely from the medication, the sedentary lifestyle of many with schizophrenia or other unknown issues is unknown. Persons with schizophrenia suffer from higher rates of diabetes with or without medication. With or without weight gain for persons taking Zyprexa or any of these medications, monitoring for cholesterol and diabetes should be done regularly. Some practitioners have used Zantac (ranitidine) type drugs to help combat the increased appetite from this medication with modest success.

Seroquel came out next. Although the usual dosage sounds higher (600 – 800mg/day), it can be equally effective. It is also approved for treatment of bipolar disorder – mania. The initial product information studies recommended that it be given twice a day, but many take it just once a day before bed. Also in the initial studies in animals, they noted cataracts in beagles, but no significant eye problem has been noted in humans. Nevertheless, evaluations for cataracts during routine eye exams is recommended. There may be less risk of EPS or weight gain with Seroquel.

The newest "typical" atypical released as of this writing is Geodon (ziprasidone). The recommended dose is 160 mg taken in divided dosages with food or all at bedtime. The body absorbs it better with food. Like Seroquel, whenever a medicine must be taken more than once a day, the likelihood of forgetting the second dose is great. (Shouldn't be a problem in group homes with paid staff, however.) Geodon is said to be the least likely to put weight on people, which is certainly a bonus. It is not without unique concerns either, however. There are multiple potential drug interactions that limit either Geodon's or the other medicines use. Initial studies felt that Geodon has the potential to alter the heart's electrical system. While current studies show no increase risk with Geodon, EKGs are a must. Actually, experience is showing that many, if not all antipsychotics could potentially alter EKG readings (specifically prolong the QTC interval, or in layman's language, too long a pause between the "lub" and "dub".) In addition, for any of these new drugs, there are also potential side effects of drowsiness, stomach upset, etc.

Abilify (aripiprazole) works quite differently from all the other newer agents. The 'partial-agonist' property means that where dopamine is excessive, Abilify blocks it—like in the pathways where hallucinations start. In the areas with too little dopamine like the movement areas, it has the potential to increase dopamine action. If experience matches theory, this agent may be a blessing for those acutely sensitive to movement disorders. It is not associated with significant weight gain or sedation. Again, we must monitor for EKG changes, and possible orthostatic hypotension (stand too quickly and get dizzy or fall). The dosage range is 10-30 mg/day.

When *The Psychiatric Tower of Babble* was written, I was on a very high soapbox decrying the use of all antipsychotic medications. I have since had to change my mind, and I got off the box.

Ross is somebody that comes to mind when I start to think negative thoughts about antipsychotic medications. Ross's mother had Rubella while pregnant with him. Although blind, functionally deaf and said to be retarded, he has many work skills. He also loves to ride a bike. When someone isn't available to be the navigator of his bike for 2, he rides the exercise bike in his home. He's ridden it so hard that the pedals came off. It was broken beyond what staff could repair. One of his jobs at work is to sort nut and bolt assemblies. He brought home a set to fix his bike. It was the wrong size. The next day, he returned the first set and brought home the correct size and fixed his bike.

Part of the reason that the exercise bike broke is that once Ross starts to do something, he does it with full force. Ross also has very severe OCD. He has destroyed hundreds of dollars of clothes in a single day when he cannot get the cloth to "line up" precisely. If shoes have a ridge out of place, he tears them. When his very heavy oak bed could not be lined up exactly in his room, he pushed it so hard it cracked. His biggest problem, however, was the fireproof door leading to his bedroom.

Since Ross and all his housemates are blind, special fire precautions in the home are mandatory. The fire codes demand this certain door remain up, and Ross demanded that it come down. Ross can't write letters to the fire marshal, so he took a more direct route. He tore the door off the hinges. Repeated doors, door -frames, behavior programs, rearrangement of rooms, etc., all ended with the same result. I watched him pull the prison-quality steel door from the frame and bend it in less than 20 seconds!

Very low doses of SSRI medication helped with the clothes compulsions, but not with the door. When the SSRI dose was increased to even a usual dosage, he became very agitated. Faced with the very real threats of the home being closed, Ross going to an institution or SOMETHING...luck prevailed. Recent information suggested that very low dosages of certain atypical antipsychotics helped with "agitation". Ross was placed on Risperdal (risperidone), two milligrams a day in addition to the SSRI and is no longer experiencing the extreme compulsive qualities (problems with clothes continue, but to a lesser extent) that he had experienced before as well as the agitation and aggression. After four years of being on these medications, the only long-term effects noted to date has been an increase in his paycheck at work. He goes by the door several times daily, and it stays put. He is no longer driven to remove it.

Given that the newer agents are so much more effective, why would any one be on the older ones? The main reasons are cost and experience in using them. In terms of cost, although the pills themselves are certainly more expensive, since the atypicals as a class have dramatically reduced hospitalization costs, improved independence and thus productivity, the cost per pill is easily outweighed. Changing someone over to the newer agents takes time, but is not undoable. On the other hand, if the older agents help.... Well...let's continue to explore the side effects of the older medications.

The most common serious side effect of any antipsychotic, but especially the older ones is tardive dyskinesia (TD). TD generally begins with movements of the tongue, mouth, and jaw. Particularly when the person is relaxed, you will notice that she looks like she is chewing a very large piece of gum. They may scrunch up their lips or smack their lips together. The person may also make a pill rolling motion with the fingers. Some people develop movement throughout their entire body.

My best friend is also a nurse. When I went into psychiatric work, she remained a 'real nurse' and worked in the hospital. She called me one day about a woman who was on an orthopedic floor (a bone floor). This elderly woman fell and broke her hip and they needed to put her in traction. Now you need to understand it had been a long time since I worked a hospital floor so I was rather curious as to why my friend would call me – from work! She informed me that this elderly lady had been on Haldol for over four decades but had not taken it for several weeks. They were wondering if the abrupt withdrawal of this medication had something to do with her fall.

After the Haldol had been abruptly stopped, this woman began to have entire body gyrations that were out of her control as a result of Tardive Dyskinesia (and possibly withdrawal dyskinesia). These gyrations caused her to fall and break her hip in the first place and were preventing her from benefiting from traction in the second place. Since this was before the days of the newer medications, she had to be placed back on even higher dosages of the Haldol until the hip could be healed. One wonders why these extreme gyrations didn't occur while the woman was on the Haldol in the first place. Her psychiatrist had noticed some mouth, lip, and tongue movements. Unfortunately, the same medications that cause the TD movements also mask it to some extent. The unplanned stopping of the medication allowed for the full display of symptoms with the tragic broken hip. At this time, many practitioners recommend Vitamin E from 400 – 1200 IU/day, sometimes with Vitamin B6 (100 mg/day) to delay or decrease the TD movements. Clozaril and some of the other atypical antipsychotics may even help treat TD.

When continuing to look at the older medications, other common side effects most associated with the high potency antipsychotics (those older antipsychotics that only require 1 to 40 mg/day to achieve the desired response) are the extrapyramidal side effects or EPS. No, the person does not develop an urge to go to Egypt and erect triangular structures. Extrapyramidal side effects are motor movement side effects.

Remember that the dopamine receptors are also located in the nervous pathways of the brain associated with movement. When the blockade affects this system, you may see more than TD including akathisia, Parkinsonism, and dystonic movements.

Have you ever been sitting at a table with one or more people who have had too much caffeine? Their legs get shaking so hard that they can literally cause the table to shake. I remember drinking so much caffeinated Diet Pepsi prior to an exam that I had an entire row of desks moving. Although I was rather impressed with my leg's abilities, the other test takers seemed less than thrilled. This is mild compared to the akathisia associated with the dopamine blockers. The person may dance from foot to foot. He may pace restlessly. The person may report feeling very anxious inside. Frequently we have misdiagnosed this restlessness as a sign that the psychotic disorder is becoming worse and medication doses are raised compounding the problem geometrically.

Interestingly, some people develop drug-induced Parkinsonism that looks like Parkinson's disease. Actual Parkinson's disease is caused from too little dopamine in the movement pathways. The person develops a mask-like facial expression that is very difficult to observe in somebody who already has a flat affect associated with schizophrenia. Other signs of Parkinsonism side effects include resting body tremors (shaking when they are relaxing, but it can go away briefly when they reach for an object, etc.), rigid posture, and a shuffling walk. While one must certainly be on the lookout for this side effect, never forget that true Parkinson's disease particularly in older people could also be present.

Dystonia often involves the muscles of the eye, neck, and/or throat. The person's eyes may move up in the socket and not come down. The neck may swell, become stiff, and even close off the airway for breathing! Dystonia looks more like an allergic reaction to the medications but is associated with the EPS movements. Dystonic reactions can be life threatening. Part of a medication history should always involve previous medications that the individual has been on. If you find out that somebody's had a dystonic reaction to a specific antipsychotic medication you certainly would never want to prescribe that same medication or one from a similar class or one runs the risk of a future dystonic reaction.

When an individual with schizophrenia has experienced EPS, particularly a dystonic reaction, the paranoia that they are already feeling as part of the illness is compounded by the body side effects that they are currently experiencing. It is often times very difficult to convince an individual with schizophrenia to go back on any sort of medication if they have experienced severe akathisia or dystonia. This is another reason for starting with the newer agents in the first place.

The EPS side effects (except TD) can be relieved by also prescribing anti-Parkinsonism medications such as benzotropine (Cogentin), amantadine (Symmetrel), diphenhydramine (Benadryl) or trihexyphenidyl (Artane). Some people have also used Inderal, the blood pressure medication, for some of the movement disorders associated with these medications. Unfortunately, these medications also have their own side effects, most notably the anticholinergic side effects that are also seen in the low potency antipsychotics (those antipsychotics that require 100 to1000 milligrams to get the desired response).

The anticholinergic side effects seen in the antiparkinsonism medications are even more commonly seen with the low potency older antipsychotics such as Thorazine and Mellaril. These side effects include impaired thinking, constipation, blurred vision, dry mouth, drowsiness, low energy, sensitivity to sun, lowered sexual drive and ability to reach orgasm, and many, many others. Some of these side effects will ease up over time or perhaps the person learns to live with feeling half dead over time. The older medications were less apt to impact on the negative symptomatology of the schizophrenia and these side effects compounded the problems and debilitated people even further.

More recently, the FDA issued a black box warning on thioridazine (Mellaril). Persons on thioridazine may experience the prolonged heart "QTc wave" interval mentioned in an earlier chapter. This too-long period between the lub and dub of the heartbeat can cause dizziness, heart problems and even death.

Since these older "major tranquilizers" can produce lethargy, drowsiness, and lack of initiative to move on with life, others have used these side effects as a desire therapeutic effect. I recently was at an inservice where a physician was describing a two-year old that was apparently "out of control". When experts couldn't think of any other options, the parents were given a bottle of liquid Mellaril, and advised to use no more than a few drops (5 to 10 mg) of the Mellaril when absolutely necessary. The parents began using over a teaspoon of Mellaril on any given day. This equated to over 25 mg of Mellaril for a two-year old child.

No one seemed concerned that the long-term ramifications of this medication could also include blindness since

Mellaril is associated with certain eye difficulties. I was aghast, but others seemed unconcerned, as the two-year old had calmed down. "Calmed down" is not a desire of treatment. The desire of treatment is increased functioning, increased participation and increased enjoyment of the world. One can calm down anyone simply with the use of anesthesia. I doubt that is being recommended in many places.

Scott brought Amanda in for a psychiatric consult. She was diagnosed with profound mental retardation, hepatitis B carrier and many, many negative behaviors. She spit. She screamed. She attacked others. She scratched herself to the point where she bled. Amanda's community doctor had been maintaining the 250-mg per day of Mellaril that she had received for years in the institutions. The new doctor questioned this practice and stopped the Mellaril at her annual physical. Unfortunately, although she was not psychotic, the Mellaril covered up some of the more noticeable symptoms of the major depression that she did have. A month later, Amanda came unglued.

Have you ever taken a non non-drowsy cold tablet (the kind that makes you sleepy) by mistake and then tried to work? That feeling of being in a cloud is what persons taking many older antipsychotic medications (and even some newer ones) often feel like. We then expect these people to go to their workshop and sort widgets by the hour. Amanda had been under this cloud for years. When the medication was abruptly stopped she experienced neuroleptic withdrawal syndrome.

The person having a massive rebound effect to their own neurotransmitters when the medications are stopped highlights neuroleptic withdrawal syndrome. The idea is that neurons which are experiencing Dopamine blockade from the antipsychotic medications adjust by becoming over sensitive to whatever dopamine they do receive. When the dopamine blockade is removed abruptly (more than 20% of the antipsychotic discontinued at a time), the receptors are freed up and react violently to all the excess dopamine. We literally create temporary illness in these people. This withdrawal phenomenon that happened to Amanda and her staff is what happened all over the country 10 – 20 years ago when systems tried to stop everyone's "behavior-control" medications.

As with Amanda, the withdrawal effect is usually not noticed right away. The antipsychotic medications often cause a person to put on excess body fat and then the medication stores itself in body fat. This fat-stored medicine is slowly used up so that you will generally not notice symptoms of withdrawal until three to four weeks later. This also explains why a person with actual schizophrenia will feel like they do not need the medicines because they can often go for days without serious problems. Unfortunately by the time the medications have slowly left their body, they have often had a major decompensation.

A common recommendation to avoid neuroleptic withdrawal syndrome particularly with thioridazine is that no more than 10 to 20 percent of the medication should be decreased every two to six months. The actual reduction process varies from person to person, and on how long they have been receiving the medications.

Oftentimes while the medications are being decreased, symptoms of the probable original psychiatric or other medical illnesses are revealed. As in Amanda's case the depression became evident. Since many people who are non-verbal act out their symptoms, you may see an increase in aggression. **THIS DOES NOT MEAN THAT YOU SHOULD ALWAYS RESTART THE ANTIPSY-CHOTIC!!!!!** It means that you should also look at the other symptoms to see what other diagnoses may be more appropriate and treat accordingly. You may see the rare person with a developmental disability experience a true psychotic decompensation with this process, but it has definitely been more the exception than the rule.

Elizabeth had been receiving over 500 mg of Thorazine a day for over 15 years. She always had problems with constipation. One day she became so constipated that she developed an obstructed bowel. The doctor in the hospital immediately discontinued the Thorazine. She was in the hospital for complications of the obstructed bowel for weeks. By the time she returned home, most of the severe withdrawal symptoms had subsided. Although it had undoubtedly been a horrendous time for her, no one wanted to restart the Thorazine. No psychiatric symptoms emerged, but staff noted that she cried more around her periods.

Medical follow up revealed that she had been suffering from very painful ovarian cysts probably for years. The first gynecologist had indicated that the cysts shouldn't be painful and felt that no treatment was warranted. When staff suggested that perhaps these same size cysts be placed on his external genitalia, another gynecologist needed to be found. The next gynecologist treated the ovarian cysts. This lady is now relaxing and enjoying a lot more of her life than she ever has.

In case you needed more reasons to avoid unnecessary medications, the older antipsychotics and potentially the newer ones as well can also cause a rare but dangerous (even fatal) side effect called Neuroleptic Malignant Syndrome (NMS). NMS is a sudden, crisis reaction to the medicines that causes extreme muscle rigidity, fever (usually over 102*F), sweating, rapid heart rate and breathing, and/or confusion. People with NMS will need to stop their medications, and a blood test for CPK enzymes MUST be done as soon as possible. Often these people are treated in an intensive care unit of the hospital. As one can see, while these medications are invaluable for the treatment of specific mental illnesses, they all carry a serious price tag of severe side effects.

Remember Charles with the sheriff's badge? As a tight-wad student having no other office than my car, Charles and I set up a plan of going out to area fast-food restaurants once a week. He always held my car door and the restaurant door. He did let me order for myself, but always insisted on carrying the tray. Somebody called

Charles chauvinistic but I loved every minute of it. He was a shy guy, but over time we developed an enjoyable camaraderie. (Although I never found illness, I certainly wasn't going to let on to my professors. These outings with Charles became the highlight of my graduate education.)

While enjoying a diet Coke at McD's (I can be tolerant of colas other than Pepsi when necessary), he told me about the night his mom's house was vandalized. I had long since realized that Charles had an absolute sense of right and wrong. There were no grays for him. It truly bothered him when anyone violated the rules. Anyway, as he told me about the break in, he related the incident like it had just happened when in fact it had occurred years before (length of time passing is a very abstract concept that is difficult for many people I work with to understand). He said the police came to the house and took a report. His mom told him, "Everything will be all right. The police took a report and that takes care of everything. Humph."

As he said that, a light went off in my head. Whenever someone in his behavioral home violated the rules - which happened quite frequently, he put on his badge and wrote a report to right the wrong. Charles had a greater grasp of reality than many people I know. He never was psychotic.

Chapter 8

The End or the Beginning?

Acts 17:18a
A group of Epicurean and stoic philosophers
began to dispute with him.
Some of them asked, "What is this babbler trying to say?"

I have met many people who are passionate for a cause. Some of my friends were part of a very successful fundraiser for cancer research after they themselves were treated for cancer or lost family members to cancer. When presenting at conferences, I meet family members of persons with disabilities and mental health difficulties who are very passionate about these issues. When recently asked why do I do the work I do, I had to admit that I started for all the wrong reasons.

I was bored. I mean, 'summer's gone on too long, there's nothing new on TV, and I miss my school friends', BORED! The year I was to start 10th grade coincided with the longest teacher's strike known to our school district. These two facts combined, resulted in such unhappiness that when I received a phone call from my youth guide at Church, I was more than glad to volunteer for just about anything. Anything, but what I got roped into. The church's nursery school was minus several key staff due to the staff's problems with the same teacher's strike (they had to stay home with their own kids!)

This unique nursery school had a director with a degree in special education (new in those days), and no place to put it to use. Since she was also the Pastor's wife, she couldn't move to a larger school district where jobs may have been available. A now local state institution (urban sprawl meets institutional outposts) still had many children with disabilities living there. A joint venture brought together children from the institution with children from the church in a not so typical preschool.

Josh, a church member's son with a disability, caused incredible stress to the program. While Josh had never been in the "Home", he had more difficulties than the "Home" kids. Following 20 months of usual development, Josh contracted viral encephalitis that left him deaf, intellectually challenged, and full of rage. Josh would not be able to attend even this pre-school until staff returned or "someone" could be found to stay with him at all times in class. I was bored. I became someone.

The first week I watched Josh run out of control, hit others, and spit. If not for a total lack of any reasonable excuses for not returning, I surely would have quit. The second week, Josh fell and skinned his knee while walking ON the climber. His silent tears were more than even I could take. I rushed over and held him in my lap. To everyone's amazement...especially my own, he stayed. When it was time for story hour, he remained in my lap and looked at the pictures. Shortly after that, he was up and running again, but at times he would stop to look for me. The next day he ran outside to play. The fact that everyone else was playing with play-doe inside was irrelevant. I stood in the doorway to keep watch over him. After about 20 minutes, he ran back to the classroom minus his shoes. I pointed down to his feet and back outside towards his shoes. In quick understanding, he ran back and got them. He even allowed me to tie them for him.

I don't remember much else about the other students, but I remember my last week with Josh. On Monday morning, Josh shocked us all. He saw me and made a flying leap for my hands. He pulled me over to a rocking chair, pushed me in it, and climbed aboard. We rocked together for over 30 minutes. All that week, this scenario played itself out again and again. I cried when the teachers' strike ended. My time with Josh ended. Although I would see him a few more times during church services, or in casual settings, our special times would never happen again. I wonder if he ever understood where I went Shortly after this, Josh's parents separated and Josh went into the foster care system. Ten years later, I broke the rules and looked for him in the state roles. I found out where he lived, but never if he was happy.

Three years later, the group home became my first "paid" job in the field of disabilities. I figured if I could handle Josh, I could handle this job. (Always hire a teenager, while she still knows everything!) While Josh had brought me to an understanding of the love, hopes, and needs in all of us, I had forgotten about him in the past few years, until someone asked how I started doing what I do. In a quick blip of brain cell retrieval, Josh's face came back to mind. Had he become one of many I would meet and forget in the line of work and service? Had my face ever come back in his memories?

I am to presume that if you've read this book this far, you either have a heart for advocacy, or my mother paid you. In either case, as Josh taught me, the time to reach out to others is NOW! The time to care is NOW! The time to let others care for you is NOW! This book is pure "babble" if the understanding of caring for all people...including their psychiatric needs is missed.

When the *Psychiatric Tower of Babble* first came out in 1996, I hoped then that parts would change with time. The use of Bible verses in this edition assures me that in 5 more years, at least those parts of this book will remain accurate. As fast as information about brain physiology is changing guarantees that aspects of this book will be obsolete perhaps before my next case of Diet Pepsi is gone. On the other hand, the on going needs for human rights, dignity, and understanding for persons with disabilities will not change. This *Quandaries* continues to look at psychiatric needs of persons with disabilities. There are many other mental health issues, however, that have not been addressed...YET! Some issues include personality disorders, Fetal Alcohol Syndrome, Autism Spectrum Disorders, substance abuse problems, etc. Stay tune for the next edition where these more specific mental health concerns will be addressed.

Joe, the man with Down syndrome (who didn't eat the beet soup either!), whose younger brother was also named Joe, was the next to teach me the lessons of love in a long line of teachers. While he never read the Bible, Joe nodded his head in agreement when he listened to the lessons in Church. When asked which was the greatest commandment in the Law. "Jesus replied: "Love the Lord your God with all your heart and with all your soul and with all your mind. This is the first and greatest commandment. And the second is like it: 'Love your neighbor as yourself.'" (Matthew 22: 36-39)

The same fall I met Josh, Joe and his life long friend Kenny had moved to the group home from the institution. Joe brought with him a paper bag full of clothes, a very used toothbrush, and a cheap, blue, wind-up alarm clock. Once settled into the group home, Joe followed the same routine morning after morning, season after season. Although Joe couldn't tell time, he valued his treasured clock in a world that had provided very little. The clock was set to go off at 6:30 AM. Joe never forgot to set his alarm clock at night for fear of not having enough time to get ready in the morning...and even more important...to help Kenny get ready in the morning. Kenny also had Down syndrome, but had more intellectual challenges than Joe. Joe had protected Kenny from the worst of the difficulties in the institution for over 3 decades. Now in this home together, Joe continued to help Kenny get up, dressed, and groomed morning after morning. Kenny relied on Joe. Joe relied on his clock.

After getting himself and Kenny ready for their days, came my favorite part of the morning. Joe never failed to stop by the doorway to the kitchen to greet me and say "I 'ike you!" Regular as clock-work, I'd respond, "I like you too." We'd both smile and continue our mornings. Like any group home staff person, besides cooking, cleaning, and dispensing unknown pills, at times I also ran errands to the store, doctor's office, etc. Joe was a frequent companion on these expeditions. One day he pointed to all the dials in my car and wanted to know what they were for. The one round 4" diameter space that was empty bothered him. I explained that it was for a clock, but my car didn't have one. In 1977, cars still needed 4" holes in the dash, not a 1" square for the LED on the radio.

The next day after a dressed Kenny was settled into his chair, Joe came by the kitchen door for his usual "I 'ike you." Instead of leaving after my response, however, he insisted that I follow him outside. Sitting on the dash of my car was a cheap, blue, wind-up alarm clock. Now I have a clock too.

References

American Psychiatric Association, (2000). *Diagnostic and Statistical Manual of Mental Disorders, 4th Edition-Text Revision.* Washington D.C.: American Psychiatric Association.

American Psychiatric Association, (2000). Practice guidelines for the treatment of patients with major depressive disorder (revision). *American journal of Psychiatry,* (157)4, supplement p. 1-6.

Antai-Otong, D., (2000). The neurobiology of anxiety disorders: implications for psychiatric nursing practice. *Issues in Mental Health Nursing,* 21, p. 71-89.

Arnold, L.E., (1993). Clinical pharmacological issues in treating psychiatric disorders of patients with mental retardation. *Annals of Clinical Psychiatry,* 51, p. 189-198.

Barnhill, l., (1999). Diagnosis and treatment of anxiety disorders in persons with developmental disabilities. *The NADD Bulletin,* (2)6, p. 110-115.

Conner, D.F., & Posever, T.A.(1998). A brief review of atypical antipsychotics in individuals with developmental disability. *Mental health Aspects of Developmental Disabilities,* (1)4, p. 93-102.

Coulter, D.L. (1993). Epilepsy and mental retardation. *American Journal on Mental Retardation, Vol. 98,* supplement, p. 1-11.

Drooker M.A. & Byck, R., (1992). Physical disorders presenting as psychiatric illness: a new view. *The Psychiatric Times,* (7), p. 19-24

Fava, M. (1997). Psychopharmacologic treatment of pathological aggression. *Psychiatric Clinics of North America* 20(2), 427-451.

Gabriel, S. (1996). *The Psychiatric Tower of Babble*. Diverse City Press: Quebec.

Gallucci, G., Buccino, D., & Cournoyer, M. (2003). Challenges related to thioridazine use in patients with mental retardation and developmental disabilities. *Mental Health Aspects of Developmental Disabilities*, (6)1, p. 21- 25.

Gedye, A, (1992). Recognizing obsessive compulsive disorder in clients with developmental disabilities. *The Habilitative Mental Healthcare Newsletter*, (11)11, p. 73-77.

Ghaemi, S., Sachs, G., Chiou, A. (1999). Is bipolar disorder still underdiagnosed? Are antidepressants overutilized? *Journal of Affective Disorders, 52*, 135-144.

Ghaziuddin, M., Alessi, N., & Greden, J. (1995). Life events and depression in children with pervasive developmental disorders. *Journal of Autism and Developmental Disorders, 25*(5), 495-502.

Globe and Mail, (2000), *Mood Disorders and Mental Health*. June 12, 2000, special supplement.

Greenberg, P., Sisitsky, T., Kessler, R., et al, (1999). The economic burden of anxiety disorders in the 1990's. *Journal of Clinical Psychiatry*, (60)7, p. 427-435.

Hales, R.E. & Yudofsky, S.C. (1999). *New Approaches to the Management of PTSD and Panic Disorder*. CME Inc, California.

Hanzel, T, Johnson, J, Harder, S., & Kalachik, J. (1999). Use of aggression to signal and measure depressive episodes within a rapid cycling bipolar disorder in an individual with mental retardation. *Mental Health Aspects of Developmental Disabilities* 2(4), 122-132.

Hellings, J. (1999). Psychopharmacology of mood disorders in persons with mental retardation and autism. *Mental Retardation and Developmental Disabilites Research reviews*, 5(4), 270-278.

Hollander, E., Dolgoff-Kaspar, B., Cartwright, C., Rawitt, R., & Novotny, S. (2001). An open trial of divalproex sodium in Autism Spectrum Disorders. *Journal of Clinical Psychiatry 62(7)*, 530-534.

Kalachnik, J., & hanzel, T., (2001). Behavioral side effects of barbiturate antiepileptic drugs in individuals with mental retardation and developmental disabilities. *The NADD Bulletin,* (4)3, p. 49-55.

Kastner, T., Walsh, K, & Fraser, M., (2001). Undiagnosed medical conditions and medication side effects presenting as behavioral/psychiatric problems in people with mental retardation. *Mental Health Aspects of Developmental Disabilities,* (4)3, p. 101-107.

King, R., (1999). Clinical implication of co-morbid bipolar disorder and obsessive compulsive disorder in individuals with developmental disabilities. *The NADD Bulletin,* (2)4, p. 63-67.

Levitas, A., Ed. (2001). A special issue: the psychiatric diagnostic interview evaluation in patients with mental retardation and developmental disabilities. *Mental Health Aspects of Developmental Disabilities,* (4)1, p. 1-48.

Levitas, A., Ed. (2001). A special issue: behavioral phenotype. *Mental Health Aspects of Developmental Disabilities*, (4)4, p. 129-165.

Lowry, M. (1997). Unmasking mood disorders: recognizing and measuring symptomatic behaviors. *The Habilitative Mental Healthcare Newsletter 16* (1), 1-6.

Lowry, M. (1998). Assessment and treatment of mood disorders in persons with developmental disabilities. *Journal of Developmental and Physical Disabilities*, 10(4), 387-406.

Lynch, C., (2000). Modifying psychotherapy for individuals with mental retardation. *The NADD Bulletin*, (3)5, p. 85-87.

Matich-Maroney, J., (2003). Mental health implications for sexually abused adults with mental retardation and developmental disabilities. *Mental health Aspects of Developmental Disabilities*, (6)1, p. 11-20.

Myers, B.A. & Pueschel, S.M., (1993). Differentiating schizophrenia from other mental and behavioral disorders in persons with developmental disabilities. *The Habilitative Mental Healthcare Newsletter*, (12)6, p. 93-98.

Myers, B. A., (1999). Psychotic disorders in people with mental retardation: diagnostic and treatment issues. *Mental Health Aspects of Developmental Disabilities*, (1)1, p. 1-11.

Medical Economics Data Production Co. (2004). *Physicians Desk Reference 54th Ed.* Montvale, NJ:Author.

National Institutes of Health (2002, July 31). NIMH study finds anti-psychotic medication useful in treating serious behavioral problems among children with Autism. Retrieved 10/5/02 from www.nih.gov/news/pr/jul2002/nimh-31.htm.

Nasrallah, H. & Smeltzer, D., (2002). *Contemporary Diagnosis and Management of the Patient with Schizophrenia.* Pennsylvania: Handbooks in Health Care Co.

Nemeroff, C., (1998). The neurobiology of depression. *Scientific American,* 6, p. 42-49.

The NIV Study Bible 10th Ed., (1995). Grand Rapids, MI: Zondervan Co.

Pary, R. Ed. (2002). A special issue: mental health problems in Down syndrome. *Mental Health Aspects of Developmental Disabilities,* (5)2, p. 33-65.

Pary, R. & Khan S. (2002). Cyclic behaviors in persons with developmental disabilities: are cluster and migraine headaches being overlooked? *Mental health Aspects of Developmental Disabilities* 5(4), 125-129.

Pary, R., Levitas, A, & Hurley, A., (1999). Diagnosis of bipolar disorder in persons with developmental disabilities. *Mental health Aspects of Developmental Disabilities,* (2)2, p. 37-49.

Poindexter, A. (1993). Can Depakote or Tegretol change my life? Behavioral consequences of simplified antiepileptic drug regimes. *The NADD Newsletter* (11)3, p. 1-3.

Pollack, M., (2001). Comorbid anxiety disorders in primary care. *Therapeutic Spotlight, supplement to Clinicians Reviews.*

Proud, H., Chard, K., Nowak-Drabik, k., & Johnson, D., (2000). Determining the effectiveness of psychotherapy with persons with mental retardation: the need to move toward empirically based research. *The NADD Bulletin,* (3)6, p. 83-86.

Reiss, S. & Aman, M.G. (eds), (1998). *Psychotropic Medication and Developmental Disabilities: The International Consensus Handbook.* Columbus, OH: The Ohio State University, Nisonger Center.

Reiss, S. & Benson, B.A. (1984). Awareness of Negative Social Conditions Among Mentally Retarded, Emotionally Disturbed Outpatients. *American Journal of Psychiatry,* (141), p. 99-90.

Reiss, S. & Benson, B.A. (1985). Psychosocial Correlates of Depression in Mentally   Retarded Adults: I. Minimal Social Supports and Stigmatization. *American Journal of Mental Deficiency,* (89) 4, p. 331-337.

Ryan, R. (1993). Medication management of post-traumatic stress disorder in persons with developmental disabilities. In *Celebrating a Decade of Excellence.* Philadelphia: 10th Annual Conference NADD, p. 1-3.

Ryan, R. & Sunada, k., (1997). Medical evaluation of persons with mental retardation referred for psychiatric assessment. *General hospital psychiatry,* (19), p. 274-280.

Sobsey, D. (1994). The research that shattered the myths: understanding the incidence and nature of abuse and abusers. *The NADD Newsletter* (11)3, p. 1-4.

Sovner R. & Hurley, A. (1983). Do the mentally retarded suffer from affective illness? *Archives of General Psychiatry, 46,* 61-67.

Sovner, R. & Hurley, A. (1989). Ten diagnostic principles for recognizing psychiatric disorders in mentally retarded persons. *Psychiatric Aspects of Mental Retardation Reviews 8*(2), 9-13.

Sovner, R. & Hurley, A. (1990). Affective disorder update. *The Habilitative Mental Healthcare Newsletter, 9,*(12), 103-108.

Sovner, R. & Pary R. (1993). Affective disorders in developmentally disabled persons. In Matson, J., 7 Barrett, R. (eds), *Psychopathology in the Mentally Retarded* (2nd Ed.), Needham Heights: Allyn & Bacon.

Stahl, S. (1999). *Psychopharmacology of Antipsychotics*. Dunitz Ltd: London.

Stahl, S. (1997). *Psychopharmacology of Antidepressants*. Dunitz Ltd: London.